MASTER
YOUR
MIND

The mind is its own place, and in itself
Can make a Heav'n of Hell, a Hell of Heav'n

– John Milton, *Paradise Lost*

MASTER
YOUR
MIND

The Mental Health Guide

Dr Neel Burton
BSc, MBBS, MRCPsych, MA (Phil), AKC

Acheron Press
Flectere si nequeo superos
Acheronta movebo

© Neel Burton 2009

Published by Acheron Press in Oxford, UK

A CIP catalogue record for this book is available from the British Library.

ISBN 978 0 9560353 1 8

Important notes from the publisher

While every effort has been made to ensure the accuracy of the information in this book, no responsibility can be accepted by the author or publisher for any loss or injury occasioned to any person acting or refraining from action as a result of this information.

This book is not intended to replace medical advice. Do consult with your doctor if you are experiencing symptoms with which you feel you need help.

Typeset by Phoenix Photosetting, Chatham, Kent, UK

Printed by Athenaeum Press Ltd, Gateshead, Tyne & Wear, UK

Contents

Introduction   1

Section 1 Mental disorders and their diagnosis   3

1   What is a mental disorder?   5
2   Anxiety disorders   8
3   Depression   18
4   Bipolar disorder   23
5   Schizophrenia   30
6   Personality disorders   40
7   Eating disorders   50
8   Alcohol or drug misuse and dependence   54
9   Receiving a diagnosis of mental disorder   59
10 Accepting a diagnosis of mental disorder   61

Section 2 Master your mind through your mind   65

11	Building confidence and self-esteem	67
12	Building relationships	72
13	Managing stress	74
14	Managing anxiety	79
15	Managing obsessions and compulsions	83
16	Fighting depression	87
17	Thinking errors in depression	90
18	Fighting thoughts of self-harm	92
19	Fighting suicidal thoughts	96
20	Improving concentration and memory	102
21	Coping with voices	106
22	Coping with delusions and hallucinations (for carers)	108
23	Coping with high expressed emotion	110
24	Coping with stigma	113
25	Preventing relapses	117
26	Aristotle on human flourishing	121

Section 3 Master your mind through your body   125

27	Monitoring your physical health	127
28	Eating healthily	129
29	Taking exercise	133
30	Sleeping well	135
31	Quitting smoking	140
32	Staying off alcohol and drugs	144

Contents

Section 4   Psychological and physical treatments   **149**

33   Psychological or 'talking' treatments   151
34   Complex Needs Service   156
35   Sedatives   158
36   Antidepressants   160
37   Mood stabilisers   165
38   Antipsychotics   172
39   Taking your medication   181
40   Electroconvulsive therapy   184

Section 5   Mental health services and the law   **187**

41   A guide to mental healthcare services   189
42   The care programme approach   198
43   The Mental Health Act   200
44   Driving and DVLA regulations   204
45   Social benefits   206
46   Advice for carers   210
47   Useful addresses   219

Introduction

There is a lot of useful advice that GPs and psychiatrists can give to their patients suffering from a mental disorder. Unfortunately, time pressures in clinical practice are such that only a small part of this knowledge can ever be imparted. I wrote this book because I didn't want so much knowledge to keep getting lost. Instead, I wanted it to be there, once and for all, in a place where anyone could find it.

Unlike many other information and self-help books, this one is specifically for people who suffer from a mental disorder, and it has been written and designed so as to be as user-friendly as possible. It is divided into a number of concise and self-contained modules, which makes it possible for you to dip in and out, and to focus on the modules that are most relevant to you at any one time. Of course, you can also read the book from cover to cover, but some people who suffer from a mental disorder may not be able to concentrate for long enough to do this.

As its name suggests, *Master your Mind* places a strong emphasis on self-help, because there really is so much that you can do to help yourself, and because self-help is simple, freely available, and – once learned – with you for always. If you suffer from a mental disorder, the information contained in this book should help you to alleviate any feelings of fear, hopeless-ness, or isolation that you may have; to take greater control of your symptoms; to make the most of the treatments and services that are available to you; and – ultimately – to improve your chances of once again leading a healthy, productive, and fulfilling life.

Neel Burton

Section 1
Mental disorders and their diagnosis

What is a mental disorder?

'Mental disorder' is difficult to define. Broadly speaking, mental disorders are psychological or behavioural patterns that involve either distress and impairment or loss of contact with reality. These experiences lie on a continuum of normal human experience, and so it is impossible to define the exact point at which they become pathological. The concept of 'mental disorder' has changed over time and across cultures, but modern classifications of mental disorders such as the *Diagnostic and Statistical Manual of Mental Disorders 4th Revision* (DSM-IV) and the *International Classification of Diseases 10th Revision* (ICD-10) are widely accepted by mental health professionals. Both ICD-10 and DSM-IV are based on scientific research and expert opinion and, particularly in the case of ICD-10, on international consultation and consensus. They list not only the different categories of mental disorder such as anxiety disorders, mood disorders, and psychotic disorders, but also the criteria according to which individual mental disorders should be diagnosed.

Mental disorders are very common. According to a World Health Organization (WHO) report, one in four people in the world will suffer from a mental health problem at some point in their life. In the UK, mental health accounts for up to one third of all general practice consultations, and every year the National Health Service (NHS) spends more money on mental healthcare than on any other area of care, including cardiovascular disease, cancer, and even primary care.

Yet mental disorders are little talked about, perhaps one of the last real taboos in modern society. This loud silence greatly contributes to the stigmatisation of people with mental disorders. As a group people with mental disorders are not unpredictable or dangerous; they are not lazy or 'moral failures'; and getting better is not simply a matter of them 'pulling themselves together'. Severe forms of mental disorder have a strong biological basis and are certainly not 'all in the mind'. For people with mental disorders, stigma can create a vicious circle of alienation and discrimination that hinders progress to recovery by promoting anxiety, depression, alcohol and drug misuse, social isolation, unemployment, homelessness, and institutionalisation. Many people with mental disorders report that the stigma that they are made to feel can be even more distressing than their symptoms; in some cases, they fear this stigma to such an extent that they are unable to accept that they are ill, and so do not seek out the help that they need.

What is a mental disorder?

Most mental disorders are eminently treatable, so obtaining help at an early stage can be of vital importance. Depending on the type and severity of symptoms, treatment and support may be provided by primary care services, by a diverse range of community mental health services, and by in-patient services. Treatment options may include medication, psychotherapy, or supportive interventions, or a combination of these. In rare cases, treatment may be provided on an involuntary basis if this is deemed to be in the best interests. In England and Wales, the Mental Health Act provides the legislative framework for providing such involuntary treatment, and similar legislative frameworks exist in Scotland, Northern Ireland, and most other countries around the world.

While mental disorders are often characterised in purely negative terms, many people with a mental disorder benefit from above-average levels of creativity, non-conformity, goal-striving, perfectionism, and empathy. Some people with a mental disorder, such as Winston Churchill (depression), Mark Twain (bipolar disorder), and John Nash (schizophrenia) have even made unique and important contributions to society.

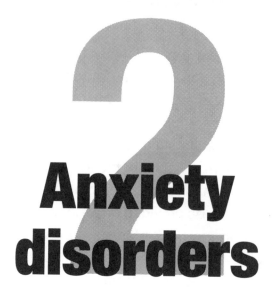

Anxiety disorders

According to its medical definition, anxiety is a state consisting of psychological and physical symptoms brought about by a sense of apprehension at a perceived threat. These psychological and physical symptoms vary greatly according to the nature and magnitude of the perceived threat, and from one person to another.

Psychological symptoms may include feelings of fear, an exaggerated startle reflex or alarm reaction, poor concentration, irritability, and insomnia. In mild anxiety, physical symptoms arise from the body's so-called fight-or-flight response, a state of high arousal that results from a surge of adrenaline. These physical symptoms include tremor, sweating, muscle tension, a fast heartbeat, and fast breathing. Sometimes people can also develop a dry mouth and the irritating feeling of having a lump in the throat.

Anxiety disorders

In severe anxiety, hyperventilation or over-breathing can lead to a fall in the concentration of carbon dioxide in the blood. This gives rise to an additional set of physical symptoms such as chest discomfort, numbness or tingling in the hands and feet, dizziness, and faintness.

Anxiety is a normal response to life experiences, a protective mechanism that has evolved both to prevent us from entering into potentially dangerous situations and to enable us to escape from them if they befall us regardless. For example, anxiety may prevent us from coming into close contact with disease-carrying or poisonous animals such as rats, snakes and spiders; from engaging with a much stronger enemy to whom we are almost sure to lose out; and even from declaring our undying love to someone who is unlikely to spare our feelings. Should we find ourselves in a potentially dangerous situation, anxiety primes our body for action and increases our performance and stamina, thereby enabling us to mount a more effective response.

Although some degree of anxiety can increase our performance on a range of tasks, *severe* anxiety can have the opposite effect and hinder our performance. Thus, whereas a confident and talented actor may perform optimally in front of a live audience, a novice may develop stage-fright and freeze. The relationship between anxiety and performance can be expressed graphically by a parabola or inverted 'U'. This is referred to as the 'Yerkes–Dodson' curve, after the psychologists RM Yerkes and JD Dodson (Figure 2.1).

According to the Yerkes–Dodson curve our performance increases with arousal but only up to a certain point, beyond

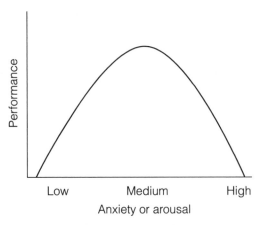

Figure 2.1 The Yerkes–Dodson curve.

which our performance begins to flag. The Yerkes–Dodson curve applies best to complex or difficult tasks, rather than to simple tasks on which the relationship between arousal and performance is more linear. The nature of the task is also important. Generally speaking, intellectually demanding tasks require a lower level of arousal for optimal performance. In contrast, tasks that call for strength and stamina require a higher level of arousal for optimal performance. This makes perfect sense given that the potentially dangerous situations that trigger a high level of anxiety are typically those that call for strength and stamina, for example, to face a foe or scamper up the nearest tree.

The Yerkes–Dodson curve suggests that very high anxiety can be more of a hindrance than a help. *From a medical standpoint, anxiety is considered to be problematic if it becomes so severe, frequent, or longstanding that it prevents a person from fulfilling his occupational or social obligations.* Such anxiety often results from an anxiety disorder, although in some instances it can also result from a number of psychiatric and medical disorders such as depression, schizophrenia, alcohol withdrawal, or an overactive thyroid gland (hyperthyroidism).

Anxiety disorders are very common and affect as many as one in every five people. They present in a number of forms, including phobic anxiety disorders, panic disorder, generalised anxiety disorder, conversion disorders, and post-traumatic stress-disorder. Phobic anxiety disorders are the most common form of anxiety disorder and involve the persistent and irrational fear of an object, activity, or situation. There are three types of phobic anxiety disorder: agoraphobia, social phobia, and specific phobias.

Phobic anxiety disorders: agoraphobia, social phobia, and specific phobias

Agoraphobia derives from the Greek 'phobia' (fear) and 'agora' (market or marketplace) and so literally means 'fear of the market place'. Contrary to popular belief agoraphobia does *not* describe a fear of open places, but a fear of places that are difficult or embarrassing to escape from, such as places that are confined, crowded, or far from home. In time, people with agoraphobia may become increasingly homebound, and may need to rely on trusted companions for their outings. A number of studies have uncovered a link between agoraphobia and poor spatial orientation, suggesting that spatial disorientation, particularly in places where visual cues are sparse, may contribute to the development of agoraphobia. Maintaining spatial orientation is clearly very important from an evolutionary standpoint, since it enables us not only to locate ourselves, but also our friends and foes, and places of water, shelter, and safety.

Social phobia refers to the fear of being judged by others and of being embarrassed and humiliated, either in most social situations or in specific social situations such as dining or public speaking. Social phobia has many features in common with shyness, and distinguishing between the two can be a cause of debate and controversy. Some critics have gone so far as to suggest that 'social phobia' is nothing more than a convenient label used to pass off a personality trait as a mental disorder, and so to legitimise its medical 'treatment'. However, social phobia is different from shyness in that it starts at a later age and is more severe and disabling. A certain degree of shyness can be an adaptive advantage, as it can protect our reputation and standing in society and prevent us from interacting too closely with potentially hostile or abusive strangers (interestingly, shyness is generally more pronounced in children and young people, no doubt because they are particularly vulnerable to potentially hostile or abusive strangers). In preventing others from hurting our feelings shyness can also protect our self-esteem, and this in turn can improve our chances of material and reproductive success.

The third and last type of phobic anxiety disorder, specific phobia, is by far the most common. Specific phobia is, as its name implies, fear of a specific object or situation. Common specific phobias involve enclosed spaces (claustrophobia), heights (acrophobia), darkness (achluophobia), storms (brontophobia), animals (zoophobia) and blood (haematophobia). Unlike other anxiety disorders, specific phobias often begin in early childhood, and there seems to be an innate predisposition to developing certain specific phobias such as phobias of spiders (arachnophobia) or snakes (ophidiophobia). Such 'biological preparedness' is intended to protect us from the potential dangers commonly faced by our ancestors, and so to increase our chances of surviving and reproducing. Today manmade dangers such as motor vehicles and electric cables are far more likely to strike us than natural dangers such as spiders and snakes, but most phobias are still of natural dangers. This may be because manmade dangers are comparatively recent arrivals and thus have not had sufficient time to imprint themselves onto the human genome.

Panic attacks and panic disorder

In a phobic anxiety disorder (whether agoraphobia, social phobia, or a specific phobia), exposure to the feared object or situation can trigger an intense attack of anxiety called a 'panic attack'. During a panic attack, symptoms are so severe that the person begins to fear that he or she is suffocating, having a heart attack, losing control, or even 'going crazy'. *He or she may develop a fear of the panic attacks themselves, and this fear in itself begins to trigger further panic attacks.* A vicious circle takes hold, with panic attacks becoming more frequent and more severe, and even occurring completely out of the blue. This pattern of panic attacks is referred to as 'panic disorder' and can in some cases lead to the development of 'secondary' agoraphobia, in which the person becomes increasingly homebound so as to minimise the risk and consequences of having a panic attack. Panic attacks can occur not only in phobic anxiety disorders but also in any anxiety disorder, depression, drug misuse, and certain physical conditions such as hyperthyroidism.

Generalised anxiety disorder

Anxiety does not invariably take a concrete form as in phobic anxiety disorders or panic disorder. In generalised anxiety disorder, anxiety is not related to any particular object or situation, but is free-floating and non-specific. There is apprehension about a number of hypothetical events that is far out of proportion to the actual likelihood or impact of those events. People with generalised anxiety disorder fear the future to such an extent they behave in a manner that is overly cautious and risk-averse; they are almost literally 'paralysed with fear'.

Obsessive-compulsive disorder (OCD)

OCD consists of predominantly obsessional thoughts, of predominantly compulsive acts or, most often, of both obsessional thoughts *and* compulsive acts. An obsessional thought is a recurrent idea, image, or impulse that is often perceived as being senseless, that is unsuccessfully resisted, and that results in marked anxiety or distress. Common obsessional thoughts involve doubt, contamination, orderliness and symmetry, safety, physical symptoms, aggression, and sex. A compulsive act is a recurrent stereotyped behavior that is not useful or enjoyable but that reduces anxiety and distress. It is often perceived as being senseless but is unsuccessfully resisted. A compulsive act may be a response to an obsessional thought or result from rules that must be applied rigidly. A typical case of obsessive-compulsive disorder is that of Mr MD:

Anxiety disorders

Mr MD is a 30-year old father of two with a nine-year history of obsessions and compulsions. He is terrified of being inadvertently responsible for harm befalling his family and so checks 'dangerous' appliances repeatedly to be sure that they are safely turned off. Over the years the doubt that he has turned off all the appliances has gradually strengthened, and simply looking at the stove is no longer reassuring enough. He must stare at each knob on the stove to make sure it is aligned in the 'off' position, and say to himself 'it's off' over and over again. Then he must place his hand on each hotplate and count to 10 to be sure that each hotplate is cold. If this ritual is interrupted, or if he loses his concentration, he has to start all over again, and it can take up to 15 minutes just to check the stove. After checking the stove he also has to check the kettle, toaster, and iron to make sure that they are all turned off and unplugged. He also checks repeatedly to make sure that all the doors and windows are locked. Getting out of the house can take up to an hour, and the rituals leave him feeling anxious and exhausted. He is constantly running late and as a result has been asked to resign from his job. Although he recognises that his rituals are senseless, he becomes extremely distressed if he tries to resist them.

– Adapted from: Clinical Research Unit for Anxiety and Depression, www.crufad.com

Conversion disorders

After a highly traumatic event such as a car crash or a physical or sexual assault, anxiety may be so sudden and overwhelming that it is converted into other symptoms. For example, anxiety may be converted into paralysis of a limb, loss of speech, or loss of vision. In some cases there may be loss of memory for the traumatic event, and the person might even depart on a sudden and unexpected journey lasting for up to several months. During this journey or 'dissociative fugue' the person is typically confused about his personal identity and may take on a separate identity. Once the journey is completed, all memory for it is typically lost. Compared to conversion disorder, dissociative fugue is very rare.

Post-traumatic stress disorder

After a highly traumatic event, anxiety can also manifest as post-traumatic stress disorder (PTSD), which is particularly common in military personnel and retired military personnel. The symptoms of PTSD include numbing, detachment, flashbacks, nightmares, partial or complete loss of memory for the traumatic event, avoidance of reminders of the traumatic event, and distress and anxiety. These symptoms may last for several years, during which associated mental disorders such as depression, other anxiety disorders, and alcohol and drug misuse may co-exist. PTSD was first recognised in the aftermath of the First World War, and its historical epithets include 'shell shock', 'combat neurosis', and 'survivor syndrome'.

Modules that should be particularly useful for people suffering from an anxiety disorder include Modules 8, 13, 14, 15, 16, 24, 31, 33, 34, 36, 37, and 42.

3
Depression

Although people colloquially use the term 'depression' to mean 'feeling sad', clinical depression is a mood disorder that, in severe cases, can lead to psychotic symptoms and even to death through self-neglect or suicide. Clinical depression (henceforth, 'depression') is very common, and is sometimes referred to as 'the common cold of psychiatry'. The symptoms of depression are often divided into three groups: core symptoms, psychological symptoms, and somatic (or physical) symptoms. These three groups of symptoms are listed in Table 3.1.

The symptoms of depression typically vary little from day to day and are unresponsive to circumstances. For example, if a person normally enjoys seeing his grandchildren, he does not lighten up even at the prospect of spending Christmas with them. Usually, symptoms have to be present for at least 14 days before a diagnosis of depression can be made, although

Table 3.1: Symptoms of depression	
Core symptoms	Low mood Loss of interest and enjoyment Fatigability
Psychological symptoms	Poor concentration Poor self-esteem Guilt Pessimism
Physical symptoms	Sleep disturbance Loss of appetite and weight loss Loss of libido Agitation or retardation (slowing down)

shorter periods may be sufficient if the symptoms are unusually severe or of rapid onset.

Mild depression is the commonest form of depression. Most people with mild depression complain of feeling low in mood and tired all the time, and sometimes also of feeling stressed or anxious. Some people instead complain that they cannot concentrate on their job or fulfil their obligations to their partner and children. Although suicidal thoughts may occur, they are usually only fleeting, and self-harm is uncommon.

Moderate depression is the classic 'textbook description' of depression that is often seen in general practice but that can be severe or persistent enough to be referred on to psychiatric services. Many if not most of the symptoms of depression (including the physical symptoms) are present to such an intense degree that the person finds it difficult if not impossible to fulfil his social obligations. Suicidal thoughts are common and may be acted upon.

Severe depression is the least common form of depression and can be described as an exaggerated form of moderate depression characterised by intense negative feelings and physical agitation or retardation. Retardation is more typical than agitation, although both may occur in the same person. In some cases, retardation may be so severe that the person is stuporous, that is, motionless, apathetic, and almost entirely unresponsive. Psychotic symptoms such as delusions and hallucinations (see Module 5, page 33) may be present in up to 25 per cent of people with severe depression, and the contents of these delusions and hallucinations are usually in keeping with a depressive outlook.

Thus delusions are commonly on the themes of guilt or poverty. Delusions of guilt involve the belief that one has committed a crime or sinned greatly, for example, by being personally responsible for an earthquake or terrorist attack that has recently been reported on the radio. Delusions of poverty involve the belief that one is financially ruined, for example, because one is being pursued by a horde of creditors or because the family house is in need of urgent and extensive repairs. Delusions may also be on a 'nihilistic' theme ('nihil' is Latin for nothing), commonly involving the belief that one is about to die or even that one is already dead. Cotard's syndrome refers to the combination of nihilistic delusions and delusions about the body ('somatic delusions'). For example, one may believe that one's guts are putrefying, or that one has lost one's blood or internal organs. Paranoid delusions, religious delusions, and delusions on other themes are also possible (see Module 5, Table 5.2).

Depression

Hallucinations are often of one or several voices, either talking to the person or about the person. The voices are often mocking or attacking, seeking to undermine the person's self-esteem or entrench existing feelings of guilt or hopelessness. Voices that order the person to do things are sometimes referred to as 'command hallucinations', and can be of particular concern if they are ordering the person to harm himself.

William Styron (1925–2006), the author of *Sophie's Choice*, wrote about his experience of severe depression in the book *Darkness Visible: A Memoir of Madness*. The following is a short extract from this book which gives a very clear idea of what severe depression can feel like.

> *In depression, this faith in deliverance, in ultimate restoration is absent. The pain is unrelenting, and what makes the condition intolerable is the foreknowledge that no remedy will come – not in a day, an hour, a month, or a minute. If there is mild relief, one knows that it is only temporary; more pain will follow. It is hopelessness even more than pain that crushes the soul. So the decision-making of everyday life involves not, as in normal affairs, shifting from one annoying situation to another less annoying – or from discomfort to relative comfort, or from boredom to activity – but moving from pain to pain. One does not abandon, even briefly, one's bed of nails, but is attached to it wherever one goes.*

What is adjustment disorder?

Adjustment disorder is a protracted response to a significant life change or life event, such as a change of job, migration, divorce, or separation. It is characterised by depressive symptoms and/or anxiety symptoms that are not severe enough to be diagnosed as either a depressive disorder or an anxiety disorder. There is usually a feeling of being unable to cope or to continue in the present situation that is accompanied by angry outbursts. Adjustment disorders are relatively short-lived and generally have a good outcome. Bereavement and psychological reactions to the onset of terminal illness are special types of adjustment disorder, although they may sometimes progress to full-scale depression.

Modules that should be particularly useful for people suffering from depression include Modules 8, 11, 12, 13, 14, 16, 17, 18, 19, 20, 21, 22, 24, 25, 26, 27, 28, 29, 30, 31, 33, 34, 37, 39, 40, and 42.

4
Bipolar disorder

Bipolar disorder or manic-depressive illness is a disorder of mood that affects about 1% of the population, and that involves recurrent episodes of abnormally elevated mood ('mania') and depression. The frequency and severity of manic and depressive episodes varies a lot from one person to another, as does the proportion of manic to depressive episodes. To meet the diagnostic criteria for bipolar disorder, a person must have had at least one episode of mania, regardless of whether he or she has ever had an episode of depression. This is because, sooner or later, an episode of depression is almost certain to supervene.

People with mania are often dressed in colourful clothing or in unusual, haphazard combinations of clothing which they complement with inappropriate accessories such as hats and sunglasses and excessive make-up, jewellery, or body art. Their behaviour is typically hyperactive, and may appear to others as being entertaining, charming, flirtatious, vigilant, assertive, or aggressive, and sometimes all of these in turn. While people with mania are typically euphoric, optimistic, self-confident, and grandiose, they may also be irritable or tearful, with rapid and unexpected shifts from one extreme to another. Their thoughts race through their mind at high speed and as a result their speech is pressured and voluble and difficult to interrupt. The author, artist, and art critic John Ruskin (1819–1900) described the experience thus: 'I roll on like a ball, with this exception, that contrary to the usual laws of motion I have no friction to contend with in my mind, and of course have some difficulty in stopping myself when there is nothing else to stop me ... I am almost sick and giddy with the quantity of things in my head – trains of thought beginning and branching to infinity, crossing each other, and all tempting and wanting to be worked out.' Sometimes their speech is so rambling or disorganised that they are unable to stick to one topic or even finish a sentence; they may ignore the strictures of grammar, step outside the confines of an English Dictionary, and even talk in rhyme and puns. An example of talking in rhymes and puns is: 'They thought I was in the pantry at home ... Peekaboo ... there's a magic box. Poor darling Catherine, you know, Catherine the Great, the fire grate, I'm always up the chimney. I want to scream with joy ... Hallelujah!'[1]. All this can make it very difficult for anyone else to be heard, let alone understood, by the person with mania.

People with mania are typically full of grandiose and unrealistic plans that they begin to act upon but soon abandon. They often

---

1 Andrew Sims, *Symptoms in the Mind: An Introduction to Descriptive Psychopathology* (1988).

engage in impulsive, pleasure-seeking, and disinhibited behaviour that may for example involve driving recklessly, taking illegal drugs, spending vast amounts of money with careless abandon, or engaging in sexual activity with near-strangers. As a result, they may end up harming themselves or others, getting into trouble with the police and authorities, or being exploited by unscrupulous individuals. People with mania may also experience psychotic symptoms such as hallucinations or delusions that make their behaviour seem all the more bizarre and out of character (see page 33). Delusional themes are usually in keeping with the elevated mood, and often involve delusions of grandeur, that is, delusions of exaggerated self-importance – of special status, special purpose, or special abilities. For example, a person with mania may believe that he is a brilliant scientist on the verge of finding a cure for AIDS, or that he is an exceptionally talented entrepreneur engaged by the Queen to rid the country of poverty. People with mania generally have very poor insight into their mental state, and typically find it very difficult to accept that they are ill. As a result, they are likely to delay getting the help that they need and, in the meantime, cause tremendous damage to their health, relationships, careers, and finances. A typical case of mania is that of Mrs AS:

> *Ten months ago Mrs AS, a community psychiatric*
> *nurse, started feeling brighter and more energetic.*
> *At work she took on many extra hours and extra*
> *roles, but to her surprise one of her colleagues*
> *reported her as unsafe. She promptly resigned*
> *claiming that she needed more time to devote*
> *to her many plans and projects. By then she*
> *couldn't stop her thoughts from racing and was*

sleeping only three or four hours a night. She rented a launderette and set out to transform it into a multipurpose centre. Then she bought three houses to rent out to the poor. She became very outgoing and acted completely out of character, dressing garishly, smoking marijuana, and getting herself arrested for being 'drunk and disorderly'. Four months ago her mood began dropping and she felt dreadful and ashamed. Today she is feeling better but has had to sell her house to pay off her debts. Her psychiatrist suggested that she start on a mood stabiliser, but she is understandably reluctant to take his advice.

In some cases a person with bipolar disorder may experience an episode of elevated mood that qualifies as hypomania rather than mania. Hypomania is a lesser degree of mania, with similar but less severe symptoms than in mania. The mood is elevated, expansive, or irritable but, in contrast to mania, there are no psychotic features and there is no *marked* impairment of social functioning. Indeed, some people with hypomania may function very effectively and be full of ideas and energy and the 'life and soul' of the party. At the same time their judgement may be subpar, and they are at an increased risk of making rash and damaging or dangerous decisions. Hypomania may herald mania, and in such cases the diagnosis simply becomes one of mania.

People who have had one or more manic episodes typically also experience episodes of depression, and sometimes also mixed episodes characterised by features of both mania *and* depression. In some cases episodes of depression in bipolar disorder can be severe, and involve both psychotic symptoms and suicidal thoughts (for more on depression, see Module 3).

Unlike conditions such as heart disease or diabetes, bipolar disorder tends to strike in the prime of life, when people are likely to be full of plans and dreams for the future. As a result of being given a diagnosis of bipolar disorder, some people may feel that all their dreams have been shattered, and that they have betrayed those that they hold most near and dear. Mixed feelings of loss, hopelessness, and guilt may exacerbate or prolong a depressive episode or give rise to further depressive episodes and, in some cases, even to thoughts of self-harm or suicide. Sadly, about 10 per cent of people with bipolar disorder go on to commit suicide. The risk of suicide is greatest during episodes of depression and mixed episodes involving both symptoms of mania and depression. Factors that are likely to increase the risk of suicide include being male, being young, being unmarried, lacking social support, having high intelligence, having high ambitions or expectations, being early in the course of the illness, having good insight into the disorder, and having recently been discharged from a psychiatric hospital. Accidents are also common in people with bipolar disorder, particularly during manic episodes when behaviour can be impulsive and reckless. For example, people with mania may get caught up in a house fire, a motoring accident, or an accidental drug overdose.

Manic and depressive episodes may last from several days to several months, and are usually separated by periods of normal mood. The length of these periods of normal mood can vary a lot from one person to another and from one period to the next. To a large extent, the goal of treatment is to extend periods of normal mood for as long as possible by stabilising mood and preventing further episodes of mood disorder. The case of Mr TP illustrates the course that bipolar disorder can take over several decades:

I have been high several times over the years, but low only once.

When I was high, I became very enthusiastic about some project or another and would work on it with determination and success. During such highs I wrote the bulk of two books and stood for parliament as an independent. I went to bed very late, if at all, and woke up very early. I didn't feel tired at all. There were times when I lost touch with reality and got carried away. At such times, I would jump from project to project without completing any, and did many things which I later regretted. Once I thought that I was Jesus and that I had a mission to save the world. It was an extremely alarming thought.

When I was low I was an entirely different person. I felt as though life was pointless and that there was nothing worth living for. Although I would not have tried to end my life, I would not have regretted death. I did not have the wish or the energy to do even the simplest of tasks. Instead I withered away my days sleeping or lying awake in bed, worrying about the financial problems that I had created

*for myself during my highs. I also had a feeling
of unreality, that people were conspiring to make
life seem normal when in actual fact it was unreal.
Several times I asked the doctor and the nurses
to show me their ID because I just couldn't bring
myself to believe that they were real.*

The initial choice of medication in bipolar disorder is principally determined by the person's current symptoms. In a manic episode the treatment most often prescribed is an antipsychotic whereas in a depressive episode it is an antidepressant, sometimes in combination with a mood stabiliser to avoid 'manic switch', that is, over-treatment into mania. Once symptoms of mania or depression have remitted, the antipsychotic or antidepressant is usually discontinued and a mood-stabiliser such as lithium is started with the aim of preventing further relapses. Lithium decreases the rate of relapse by about one-third, but is more effective against mania than against depression. It is also the only mood stabiliser that has been proven to reduce the risk of suicide. For further information on antipsychotics, antidepressants, and mood stabilisers, see Modules 37–39.

Modules that should be particularly useful for people suffering from bipolar disorder include Modules 8, 9, 10, 11, 12, 13, 14, 16, 17, 18, 19, 20, 21, 22, 24, 25, 26, 27, 28, 29, 30, 31, 32, 33, 37, 38, 39, 40, 42, and 44.

5

Schizophrenia

The term 'schizophrenia' was coined in 1910 by the Swiss psychiatrist Paul Eugen Bleuler (1857–1939) and is derived from the Greek words 'schizo' (split) and 'phren' (mind). Although people often mistakenly think of schizophrenia as a 'split personality', Bleuler had actually intended the term to refer to a 'loosening' or 'opening up' of thoughts and feelings.

Robert Louis Stevenson's novel *The Strange Case of Dr Jekyll and Mr Hyde* did much to popularise the concept of a 'split personality', sometimes also referred to as 'multiple personality disorder'. However, multiple personality disorder is a vanishingly rare condition that is totally unrelated to schizophrenia; the vast majority of psychiatrists have never seen a case of multiple personality disorder, and many think that the condition does not even exist. Although people with schizophrenia may hear voices or have strange beliefs that seem out of keeping with their usual selves, this is not the same as having a 'split personality'. Unlike Dr Jekyll, people with schizophrenia do not suddenly change into a different, unrecognisable person.

Although the term 'schizophrenia' has lead to much confusion about the nature of the disorder, Bleuler had intended it to replace the older, even more misleading term of 'dementia praecox' ('dementia of early life'). This term had been championed by the German psychiatrist Emil Kraepelin (1856–1929) who mistakenly believed that the disorder occurred only in young people and that it inevitably led to mental deterioration. Bleuler disagreed on both counts and, in an attempt to clarify matters, changed the name of the disorder to 'schizophrenia'. He believed that, contrary to leading to mental deterioration, schizophrenia led to a sharpening of the senses and to a heightened consciousness of experiences and memories.

Although Kraepelin may have had some mistaken beliefs about the nature of schizophrenia, he is generally credited as being the first person to isolate it from other forms of psychosis, and in particular from the 'affective psychoses' that occur in mood disorders such as mania and depression. Kraepelin first 'discovered' schizophrenia in 1887, but recently uncovered evidence seems to suggest that schizophrenia is as old as mankind itself.

Unfortunately, many people with schizophrenia and their families do not talk openly about their plight for fear of being misunderstood or stigmatised. This deplorable state of affairs can lead to the impression that schizophrenia is rare. In fact, the chance of any given person developing schizophrenia in his lifetime is about 1 per cent, and most people will know of at least someone with the disorder. Schizophrenia can present at any age, but it typically presents in early adulthood and is rare in childhood and early adolescence. Unlike anxiety and depressive disorders which tend to be more common in women, schizophrenia affects men and women in more or less equal numbers. However, the disorder tends to present at a younger age in men, and to affect them more severely. Schizophrenia exists in all societies, all cultures, and all ethnicities, but it has been found to be more common in inner cities and urban areas than in rural areas. The reasons for this are unclear: it could be that the stress of urban living increases the risk of the disorder, or that people with the disorder have an overall tendency to migrate out of rural areas and into urban ones. Interestingly, the outlook for people with schizophrenia is generally more favourable in traditional societies than in modern societies. This may be because people in traditional societies are more tolerant of mental disorder and better able to pull together and support mentally disordered members of their community.

The symptoms of schizophrenia are numerous, and present in such a variety of combinations and severities that it is impossible to describe 'a typical case of schizophrenia'. In the short term, symptoms may wax and wane, with the person experiencing both good days and bad days. In the long term, the emphasis may shift from one group of symptoms to another, presenting different challenges for the person and his or her carers. The symptoms of schizophrenia are usually divided into three groups: positive symptoms, cognitive symptoms, and negative symptoms, as listed in Table 5.1.

Table 5.1: Symptoms of schizophrenia	
Positive symptoms	Delusions ⎫ Hallucinations ⎭ Psychotic symptoms
Cognitive symptoms	Difficulties with attention, concentration, and memory
Negative symptoms	Restricted amount and/or range of thought and speech Restricted range of emotions, or inappropriate emotions Loss of drive and motivation Social withdrawal

The *positive symptoms* of schizophrenia consist of hallucinations and delusions which are usually as real to the person with schizophrenia as they are unreal to everybody else. Positive symptoms are usually considered to be the hallmark of the disorder, and they are often most prominent in its early stages. They are often precipitated by stressful situations such as breaking off a relationship, leaving home to go to university, or taking drugs (a form of biological, as opposed to psychological, stress).

Psychiatrists define a hallucination as a 'sense perception that arises in the absence of a stimulus'. Hallucinations can involve hearing, seeing, smelling, tasting or feeling things that are not actually there; in schizophrenia they most commonly involve hearing voices. These voices can either speak directly *to* the person with schizophrenia (second-person – 'you' – voices) or *about* him (third-person – 'he' or 'she' – voices). Voices are often intensely distressing, particularly if they involve threats or abuse, or if they are loud and incessant. One might begin to experience something of this distress by turning on both the radio and the television at the same time, both at full volume, and then trying to hold a normal conversation. While voices are often distressing, they are not necessarily so. Some people with schizophrenia may get used to their voices and even begin to experience them as a source of comfort and reassurance. This is especially likely if the voices are those of old acquaintances, dead ancestors, or 'guardian angels'.

Delusions are defined by psychiatrists as 'strongly held beliefs that are not amenable to logic or persuasion and that are out of keeping with their holder's background or culture'. Although delusions are not necessarily false, the process by which they are arrived at is usually bizarre and illogical. In schizophrenia, delusions most often involve being persecuted, controlled, or 'referenced', although they can also be along other so-called 'delusional themes'. Common delusional themes and some examples of each are listed in Table 5.2.

As positive symptoms correspond to the general public's idea of 'madness', people with prominent positive symptoms may evoke feelings of fear and anxiety in others. Such feelings are often reinforced by selective reporting in the media of the rare headline tragedies involving people with (usually untreated) mental disorder. The reality is that the vast majority of people with schizophrenia are no more likely than the average person to pose a risk to others, but far more likely than the average person to pose a risk to themselves. For example, they may neglect their safety and personal care or leave themselves open to emotional, physical, or financial exploitation.

Table 5.2: Delusional themes	
Delusions of persecution	Delusions of being persecuted – for example, being spied upon by secret services or being poisoned by aliens
Delusions of control	Delusions that one's feelings, thoughts, or actions are being controlled by an external force – for example, having one's thoughts 'stolen' by aliens and replaced by different thoughts
Delusions of reference	Delusions that objects, events, or other persons have a particular and unusual significance relating to oneself – for example, receiving a series of coded messages from the aliens while listening to a radio programme
Delusions of grandeur	Delusions of being invested with special status, a special purpose, or special abilities – for example, being the most intelligent person on earth and having the responsibility of saving it from climate change. Delusions of grandeur are more common in manic psychosis than in schizophrenia
Religious delusions	Delusions of having a special relationship with God or a supernatural force – for example, being the next Messiah, or being persecuted by the Devil
Delusions of guilt	Delusions of having committed a crime or having sinned greatly – for example, being personally responsible for a recent terrorist attack and thus deserving of severe punishment
	continued overleaf

Table 5.2: Delusional themes – *contd*	
Nihilistic delusions	Delusions that one no longer exists or that one is about to die or suffer a personal catastrophe. In some cases there may be a belief that other people or objects no longer exist or that the world is coming to an end. Nihilistic delusions are more common in depressive psychosis than in schizophrenia
Somatic delusions	Delusions of being physically ill or of having deformed body parts
Delusions of jealousy	Delusions that one's spouse or partner is being unfaithful. Delusions of jealousy are sometimes referred to as 'Othello syndrome'
Delusions of love	Delusions of being loved by someone who is inaccessible or with whom one has little contact
Delusions of misidentification	Delusions that familiar people have been replaced by identical-looking imposters (Capgras delusion), or that they are disguised as strangers (Fregoli delusion)

Cognitive symptoms involve difficulties with concentration and memory that can cause difficulty registering and recalling information, thinking and expressing thoughts, and understanding conversation. Cognitive symptoms are often detectable in the so-called 'prodromal phase' of schizophrenia, before the onset of positive symptoms. While they are often less evident than positive symptoms, cognitive symptoms can be just as distressing and disabling.

Whereas positive symptoms can be thought of as an excess or distortion of normal functions, *negative symptoms* can be thought of as a diminution or loss of normal functions. Compared with positive symptoms, negative symptoms tend to be more subtle and less noticeable, but also more persistent and more pervasive (affecting several areas of functioning). In some cases they may dominate the clinical picture, but in others they may be altogether absent. At times they can persist even throughout periods of remission, long after any positive symptoms have burnt out or faded into the background. During these periods of remission, the extent of any residual negative symptoms is an important determinant of the person's ability to function and, so, of his or her quality of life. Negative symptoms can be difficult to pinpoint and are often misconstrued by the general public – and sometimes also by relatives and carers – as laziness or obstreperousness rather than as the symptoms of a mental disorder. For psychiatrists, negative symptoms can sometimes be difficult to distinguish from the symptoms of depression, which is common in people with schizophrenia, or from some of the side-effects of antipsychotic medication. Negative symptoms respond poorly to antipsychotic medication, and their treatment often presents a difficult challenge.

The course of schizophrenia can vary considerably from one person to the next, but it is often marked by a number of distinct phases. In the acute ('initial and short-lasting') phase, positive symptoms come to the fore, while any cognitive and negative symptoms that may already be present appear to sink into the background. The person with schizophrenia typically reaches a crisis point when contact with mental health services is made. Antipsychotic medication is started and the acute phase resolves, although residual symptoms can remain in the background for some time. As the acute phase resolves, cognitive and negative symptoms may start to dominate the picture. This chronic (or 'long-lasting') phase, if it occurs, may last for a period of months or even several years. It may be punctuated by relapses to the acute phase, which are commonly precipitated by stressful life events, reduction or discontinuation of antipsychotic medication, or alcohol or drug misuse. Complete recovery from schizophrenia is possible, but most often the illness runs a long-term course punctuated by episodes of relapse and remission. Overall, the average life expectancy of people with schizophrenia is reduced by 10 to 12 years, owing to increased physical health problems, increased risk of accidents, and a high suicide rate. Sadly, about 10 per cent of people with schizophrenia eventually commit suicide. Risk factors for suicide include being young, being male, being early in the course of the disorder, having good insight into the disorder, coming from a high socioeconomic family background, having high intelligence, having high expectations, being unmarried, lacking social support, and being recently discharged from hospital.

The case of Valerie is typical of the acute phase of schizophrenia when positive symptoms come to the fore and a crisis point is reached when contact with psychiatric services is made:

> *Valerie is a 23-year-old anthropology student from Australia who shares a house with three other students on her course. Her housemates report that for the past six months Valerie has been behaving oddly and that since the beginning of term four weeks ago she has not attended a single lecture. One month ago, she received a phone call to tell her that her closest childhood friend, Chloe,*

had died in a motorbike accident. Since then, Valerie has been locking herself in her room for increasing amounts of time, banging on the furniture and apparently shouting to herself. Her housemates eventually persuaded her to see a general practitioner.

When Valerie arrived at the surgery, she was so agitated and distressed that she could not reply to most of the doctor's questions. However, the doctor was able to make out that Valerie was hearing three or four male voices coming from outside her head: the voices were talking together about her, making fun of her, blaming her for her family's financial problems, and commenting on her thoughts and actions. According to Valerie, they were the voices of SAS paratroopers who had been engaged by her parents to destroy her by putting harmful thoughts, such as the thought of cutting her wrists, into her head.

Towards the end of the consultation, when the doctor stood up to hold the door open for her, Valerie screamed, 'I've seen your belt, they've sent you, they've sent you to distract me. I can't ... I can't fight them anymore!' and ran out to the reception area.

Modules that should be particularly useful for people suffering from schizophrenia include Modules 8, 9, 10, 11, 12, 13, 14, 16, 17, 18, 19, 20, 21, 22, 23, 24, 25, 28, 29, 30, 31, 32, 33, 34, 39, 42, and 44.

---

6 Personality disorders

The study of human personality or 'character' dates back at least to antiquity. In his *Characters*, Tyrtamus (371–287 BC) – nicknamed 'Theophrastus' or 'divinely speaking' by his contemporary Aristotle – divided the people of the Athens of the fourth century BC into 30 different personality types. The *Characters* exerted a strong influence on subsequent studies of human personality such as those of Thomas Overbury (1581–1613) in England and Jean de la Bruyère (1645–1696) in France.

The concept of personality disorder itself is much more recent, and tentatively dates back to the French psychiatrist Philippe Pinel's 1801 description of *manie sans délire*, a condition which he characterised as outbursts of rage and violence ('manie') in an absence of any signs of psychotic illness such as delusions and hallucinations ('délires'). About 60 years later, in 1896, the German psychiatrist Emil Kraepelin (1856–1926) described seven forms of antisocial behaviour under the umbrella of 'psychopathic personality'. This term was later broadened by Kraepelin's younger colleague Kurt Schneider (1887–1967) to include those who 'suffer from their abnormality'. Schneider's seminal volume, *Psychopathic Personalities* (1923), still forms the basis of current classifications of personality disorders such as that contained in the American classification of psychiatric disorders, the Diagnostic and Statistical Manual of Mental Disorders 4th Revision (DSM-IV).

Today DSM-IV defines a personality disorder as an enduring pattern of inner experience and behaviour that deviates markedly from cultural expectations, is inflexible and pervasive, has its onset in adolescence or early adulthood, is stable over time, and leads to distress or impairment. DSM-IV lists ten personality disorders, and allocates each one to one of three groups or 'clusters': A, B, or C (Table 6.1).

Before going on to characterise these ten personality disorders, it is important to remember that they are more the product of historical observation than of scientific study, and thus that they are rather vague and imprecise concepts. For this reason, they rarely present in their pure 'textbook' form, and have a marked tendency to blur into one another. Their division into three clusters (A, B, and C) in DSM-IV is intended to reflect this tendency, with a given personality disorder most likely to blur with other personality disorders within its own cluster (Table 6.1).

The majority of people with a personality disorder never come into contact with psychiatric services, and those who do usually do so in the context of another psychiatric disorder or at a time of personal crisis, for example, after harming themselves

Table 6.1: DSM-IV classification of personality disorders		
Cluster	Description	Personality disorders in the cluster
A	Odd, bizarre, eccentric	Paranoid Schizoid Schizotypal
B	Dramatic, erratic	Antisocial Borderline Histrionic Narcissistic
C	Anxious, fearful	Avoidant Dependent Obsessive–compulsive (Anankastic)

or committing a criminal offence. Nevertheless, personality disorders are important to psychiatrists and doctors in general because they predispose to mental disorders and affect the presentation and treatment of mental disorders that are already present. They also (by definition) result in considerable distress and impairment, and may therefore need to be addressed 'in their own right'.

Paranoid personality disorder

Cluster A comprises paranoid, schizoid, and schizotypal personality disorder. Paranoid personality disorder is characterised by a pervasive distrust of others, including even friends and partner. The person is guarded and suspicious, and constantly on the lookout for clues or suggestions to confirm his or her fears. He or she has a strong sense of self-importance and personal rights, is overly sensitive to setbacks and rebuffs, easily feels shame and humiliation, and persistently bears grudges. As a result he or she may have a tendency to withdraw from other people, and find it particularly difficult to engage in close relationships.

Schizoid personality disorder

Coined by Bleuler in 1908, the term 'schizoid' designates a natural tendency to direct attention toward one's inner life and away from the external world. In schizoid personality disorder, the person is detached and aloof and prone to introspection and fantasy. He or she has no desire for social or sexual relationships, is indifferent to others and to social norms and conventions, and lacks emotional response; in extreme cases, he or she may appear cold and callous. Treatment is often not provided because people with schizoid personality disorder are generally able to function well despite their reluctance to form close relationships, and are not unduly concerned by the fact that they may be seen to have a mental disorder. Another view about people with schizoid personality disorder is that they are highly sensitive and have a rich inner life; while they experience a deep longing for intimacy, they find initiating and maintaining interpersonal relationships too difficult or too distressing and so retreat into their inner worlds.

Schizotypal disorder

Schizotypal disorder is characterised by oddities of appearance, behaviour, and speech, and anomalies of thinking similar to those seen in schizophrenia. Anomalies of thinking may include odd beliefs, magical thinking (for example, thinking that words affect the world – 'speak of the devil and he'll appear'), suspiciousness, obsessional ruminations, and unusual perceptual experiences. A person with schizotypal disorder often fears social interaction and sees other people as ill-intentioned and potentially harmful. This may lead him or her to develop so-called 'ideas of reference', which are fleeting impressions that objects, people, or situations have a special significance for him or her. For example, he or she may have the impression that strangers on the bus are talking about him or her, or that the traffic warden's signaling is an elaborate means of revealing his or her destiny. Compared to the average person, people who suffer from schizotypal disorder have a relatively high probability of 'converting' to schizophrenia at some time in the future; for this reason, schizotypal disorder has historically been referred to as 'latent schizophrenia'.

Antisocial personality disorder

Cluster B comprises antisocial, borderline, histrionic, and narcissistic personality disorder. Until Schneider broadened the concept of personality disorder to include those who 'suffer from their abnormality', personality disorder was more or less synonymous with antisocial personality disorder. Antisocial personality disorder is far more common in men than in women, and is characterised by a callous unconcern for the feelings of others. The person disregards social rules and obligations, is irritable and aggressive, acts impulsively, lacks guilt, and fails to learn from experience. In many cases he has no difficulty finding relationships, and can even appear superficially charming (the so-called 'charming psychopath'). However, his relationships are usually fiery, turbulent, and short-lived. People with antisocial personality disorder often have a criminal record or even a history of being in and out of prison.

Borderline personality disorder

In borderline personality disorder, the person essentially lacks a sense of self, and as a result experiences feelings of emptiness and fears of abandonment. There is a pattern of intense but unstable relationships, emotional instability, outbursts of anger and violence (especially in response to criticism), and impulsive behaviour. Suicidal threats and acts of self-harm are common, for which reason people with borderline personality disorder frequently come into contact with general practitioners, A&E doctors, and psychiatrists. Borderline personality disorder was so-called because it was thought to lie on the 'borderline' between neurotic (anxiety) disorders and psychotic disorders such as schizophrenia and bipolar affective disorder. It has been suggested that borderline personality disorder often results from childhood sexual abuse, and that the reason why it is more common in women is because women are more likely to be victims of childhood sexual abuse. However, feminists have argued that borderline personality disorder merely *appears* to be more common in women, since women presenting with angry and promiscuous behaviour tend to be diagnosed with borderline personality disorder, whereas men presenting with identical behaviour tend to be diagnosed with antisocial personality disorder.

Histrionic personality disorder

People with histrionic personality disorder lack a sense of self-worth, for which reason they depend on the attention and approval of others. They often seem to be dramatising or 'playing a part' ('histrionic' derives from the Latin 'histrionicus', 'pertaining to the actor') in a bid to attract and manipulate attention. They may take great care of their physical appearance and behave in a manner that is overly charming or inappropriately seductive. As they crave excitement and act on impulse or suggestion, they may put themselves at risk of having an accident or being exploited. Their dealings with other people often seem insincere or superficial, which can impact on their social and romantic relationships. This is especially distressing for them, because they are especially sensitive to criticism and rejection and react badly to loss or failure.

Narcissistic personality disorder

Narcissistic personality disorder takes its name from the myth of Narcissus, a beautiful youth who fell in love with his own reflection. In narcissistic personality disorder the person has a grandiose sense of self-importance, a sense of entitlement, and a need to be admired. He is envious of others and expects them to be the same of him. He lacks empathy and readily exploits others to achieve his goals. To others he may seem self-absorbed, controlling, intolerant, selfish, and insensitive. If he feels slighted or ridiculed, he may be provoked into a fit of destructive anger and revenge-seeking. Such 'narcissistic rage' can have dire consequences for all those involved.

Avoidant personality disorder

Cluster C comprises avoidant, dependent, and anankastic personality disorder. In avoidant personality disorder, the person is persistently tense because he or she believes that he or she is socially inept, unappealing, or inferior, and as a result fears being embarrassed, criticised, or rejected. He or she avoids meeting people unless he or she is certain of being liked, is restrained even in his or her intimate relationships, and avoids taking risks. Avoidant personality disorder is strongly associated with anxiety disorders, and may also be associated with actual or perceived rejection by parents or peers during childhood.

Dependent personality disorder

Dependent personality disorder is characterised by a lack of self-confidence and an excessive need to be taken care of. The person needs a lot of help to make everyday decisions and needs important life decisions to be taken for him or her. He or she greatly fears abandonment and may go through considerable lengths to secure and maintain relationships. A person with dependent personality disorder sees him- or her-self as inadequate and helpless, and so abdicates personal responsibility and puts his or her fate in the hands of one or more protective others; he or she imagines being at one with these protective others whom he or she idealises as being competent and powerful, and towards whom he or she behaves in a manner that is ingratiating and self-effacing. People with dependent personality disorder often assort with people with a cluster B personality disorder, who feed from the unconditional high-regard in which they are held.

Anankastic personality disorder

Anankastic personality disorder is characterised by excessive preoccupation with details, rules, lists, order, organisation, or schedules; perfectionism so extreme that it prevents a task from being completed; and devotion to work and productivity at the expense of leisure and relationships. A person with anankastic personality disorder is typically doubting and cautious, rigid and controlling, humorless, and miserly. His or her underlying high level of anxiety arises from a perceived lack of control over a universe that escapes his or her understanding. As a natural consequence, he or she has little tolerance for grey areas and tends to simplify the universe by seeing actions and beliefs as either absolutely right or absolutely wrong. His or her relationships with friends, colleagues, and family tend to be strained by the unreasonable and inflexible demands that he or she makes upon them.

Personality disorders

Modules that should be particularly useful for people suffering from a personality disorder include Modules 1, 8, 11, 12, 13, 16, 17, 18, 19, 28, 29, 30, 31, 32, 33, 34, 35, and 42.

7

Eating disorders

Anorexia nervosa is particularly common in adolescent girls and young women, although it can also occur in older age groups and in men. It is characterised not only by an abnormally low body weight, but also by a disturbed perception of body weight or shape, and by an intense fear of gaining weight or becoming fat. Weight may be lost through food restriction or excessive exercise and, in some cases, also by self-induced vomiting or the misuse of diuretics, laxatives, enemas, and stimulant drugs. A person with suspected anorexia nervosa needs to come to urgent medical attention because he or she is at a high risk of serious medical complications, and because a number of serious psychiatric and medical disorders (such as depressive disorder, obsessive-compulsive disorder, schizophrenia, diabetes mellitus, hyperthyroidism, and Crohns's disease) can present just like anorexia nervosa, and so need to be either excluded or diagnosed and treated. Some of the medical complications of anorexia nervosa are listed in Table 7.1.

The management of anorexia nervosa depends on its severity. It is important to agree a realistic treatment plan, aiming for a balanced diet of about 3000 kcal a day provided as small meals and supplementary snacks. Talking treatments such as supportive therapy or cognitive-behavioural therapy can help to alter disturbed perceptions of the body, and family therapy can help to alleviate tensions in the family. Physical and mental health should be monitored at regular intervals so that any medical complications or associated psychiatric disorders such as

Table 7.1: Some of the medical complications of anorexia nervosa

Dehydration
Life-threatening electrolyte disturbances
Arrhythmias (abnormal heart rhythms)
Heart failure
Seizures
Vitamin deficiencies
Anaemia
Erosion of tooth enamel from self-induced vomiting
Constipation
Peptic ulceration (ulceration of the stomach lining)
Pancreatitis (inflammation of the pancreas)
Kidney stones
Kidney failure
Amenorrhoea (loss of menstrual periods)
Osteoporosis
Muscle cramps
Peripheral neuropathy (loss of sensation in the hands and feet)
Dry skin
Brittle hair and nails
Increased susceptibility to infections

anxiety or depression can be detected early and treated. Hospitalisation may be required in severe cases, especially in the presence of medical complications or associated psychiatric disorders. Unfortunately, the long-term mortality rate is around 15% – higher than in any other mental disorder.

Like anorexia nervosa, bulimia nervosa is more common in women than in men, and more common in industrialised societies that idealise thinness and beauty. Bulimia nervosa is characterised by recurrent episodes of binge-eating followed by attempts to counteract the 'fattening' effect of the food by self-induced vomiting, prolonged fasting, excessive exercise, or the misuse of diuretics, laxatives, enemas, or stimulant drugs. Although the person's self-evaluation is unduly influenced by body weight and shape, he or she is usually of normal weight. However, attempts to counteract binges can lead to serious medical complications including drug overdose, dehydration, electrolyte abnormalities, cardiac arrhythmias (abnormal heart rhythms), and seizures. In terms of management, talking treatments such as supportive therapy or cognitive-behavioural therapy can help to alter disturbed perceptions of the body. Physical and mental health should be monitored at regular intervals so that any medical complications or associated psychiatric disorders such as anxiety or depression can be detected early and treated. Hospitalisation may be required in severe cases, especially in the presence of medical complications or associated psychiatric disorders. Serotonin selective reuptake inhibitors (SSRIs, see Module 37 on antidepressants) have been demonstrated to have a specific anti-bulimic effect at higher doses, and they are sometimes prescribed to people with bulimia nervosa. The prognosis or outcome of bulimia nervosa is generally more favourable than that of anorexia nervosa, not least because people with bulimia nervosa are more keen to seek and accept help.

Modules that should be particularly useful for people suffering from an eating disorder include Modules 8, 11, 12, 13, 14, 16, 17, 18, 19, 28, 29, 33, 34, 37, and 42

Alcohol or drug misuse and dependence

According to national guidelines, men should drink no more than 21 units of alcohol a week, and no more than four units in any one day. Women should drink no more than 14 units of alcohol a week, and no more than three units in any one day. Beyond this there appears to be an increasing risk of alcohol-related health and social problems.

One unit is about 8g of alcohol, equivalent to half a pint of ordinary beer, one glass of table wine, one conventional glass of sherry or port, or one single measure of spirits. One bottle of wine is equivalent to approximately 12 units, and one bottle of spirits to approximately 40 units.

The following are some of the features of alcohol dependence. Only some of these features need to be present for a confident diagnosis of alcohol dependence to be made.

Alcohol or drug misuse and dependence

- There is a strong compulsion to drink.

- Drinking begins taking priority over other activities.

- Drinking becomes more stereotyped, that is, more patterned and routine.

- There is increased tolerance to drink, meaning that increasing amounts of drink are needed to produce the same effect.

- There are repeated withdrawal symptoms.

- These withdrawal symptoms are relieved through more drinking.

- Attempts at quitting drink have so far been unsuccessful.

Alcohol dependence is fairly common, affecting about 7% of all men and 2% of all women in the UK. However, heavy drinking and hazardous drinking are even more common. Although alcohol misuse is most prevalent among young men, in recent years there has been a disproportionate rise in the numbers of women and teenagers misusing alcohol. Unfortunately, women have a stronger genetic predisposition to alcohol dependence and are also more likely to suffer from its physical complications.

Withdrawal symptoms usually occur after several years of heavy drinking and range from mild anxiety and sleep disturbance to life-threatening delirium tremens. Symptoms are most likely to occur first thing in the morning, and commonly include agitation, tremor ('the shakes'), sweating, nausea, and retching. If these symptoms are not relieved by alcohol or medical treatment, they may last for several days and progress to include perceptual distortions and hallucinations and delirium tremens, a delirious disorder characterised by, among others, fear and agitation, vivid hallucinations and delusions, coarse tremor, nausea and vomiting, and seizures.

Some of the other complications of alcohol misuse are listed in Table 8.1.

Table 8.1: Some of the complications of alcohol misuse	
Psychiatric	Mood and anxiety disorders Suicide and deliberate self-harm Short-term amnesia (memory impairment) Alcoholic dementia Sexual problems: decreased libido and impotence Pathological jealousy Alcoholic hallucinosis (auditory hallucinations)
Neurological	Seizures Delirium tremens Wernicke–Korsakov syndrome (memory loss and other symptoms) Peripheral neuropathy (loss of sensation in the hands and feet)
Gastrointestinal	Oesophageal varices that can cause fatal bleeding Gastritis Peptic ulceration (ulceration of the stomach lining) Pancreatitis (inflammation of the pancreas) Alcoholic hepatitis Cirrhosis Cancer of the oesophagus, stomach, and liver

Table 8.1: Some of the complications of alcohol misuse – *contd*	
Cardiovascular	High blood pressure Cardiac arrhythmias (abnormal heart rhythms) Cardiomyopathy (disease of the heart muscle)
Other	Hypoglycaemia Vitamin deficiencies Anaemia Accidents, especially head injury Hypothermia Respiratory depression Increased susceptibility to infections Foetal alcohol syndrome

In addition to these psychiatric and physical complications, alcohol can also cause a number of social complications such as family and marital difficulties, employment difficulties, accidents, financial problems, and crime and related legal problems.

Drug misuse can lead to similar social problems. Intravenous drug misuse carries a risk of local complications such as infection of the injection site, and systemic complications such as HIV and hepatitis B and C. Drug misuse in early pregnancy can lead to foetal abnormalities and, in late pregnancy, to dependence in the foetus. Psychiatric disorders such as depressive disorders, anxiety disorders, and personality disorders are common in drug users, and are often precipitated or perpetuated by drug misuse.

Opioid drugs such as heroin and morphine are particularly dangerous. This is because tolerance develops rapidly, but falls off soon after the drug is stopped. *This may lead to a fatal over-*

dose if the drug is restarted at the same (high) dose. The opioid withdrawal syndrome is very unpleasant, and includes intense craving, as well as symptoms such as sweating, restlessness, muscle pains, abdominal cramps, vomiting, and diarrhoea. These symptoms begin about 4–6 hours after the last dose, peak at 24–48 hours, and subside over 7–10 days.

Stimulant drugs such as cocaine and amphetamines may result in disinhibited and aggressive behaviour and in psychotic symptoms similar to those experienced in mania or schizophrenia. Overdose can lead to tremor, confusion, seizures, stroke, cardiac arrhythmias (abnormal heart rhythms), myocardial infarction (heart attack), and respiratory arrest. The withdrawal syndrome is marked by intense craving, as well as symptoms such as anxiety, low mood, tiredness, and bad dreams.

Benzodiazepines are prescription medicines that are used as sedatives and that are often misused. Tolerance develops rapidly, and ever increasing doses are needed to produce the same effect. *Accidental overdose is easy to come by, as benzodiazepines have additive effects with other drugs such as opioids and alcohol.* Overdose can lead to coma and death. Dependence is common, and the withdrawal syndrome consists of symptoms such as anxiety, irritability, tremor, and disturbed sleep.

For advice on the management of alcohol or drug misuse and dependence, see Module 33.

Modules that should be particularly useful for people with alcohol or drug misuse or dependence include Modules 11, 12, 13, 14, 16, 17, 18, 19, 28, 29, 30, 31, 32, 33, 34, 35, 36, and 42.

Receiving a diagnosis of mental disorder

The majority of medical conditions are defined either by their cause ('aetiology') or by the damage to the body ('pathology') that they result from, and for this reason are relatively easy to define and recognise. For example, malaria is caused by protozoan parasites of the genus *Plasmodium*, and cerebral infarction ('stroke') results from the obstruction of an artery in the brain. Unfortunately mental disorders cannot as yet be defined by their aetiology or pathology, and so must be defined according to their clinical manifestations or symptoms. Thus, a psychiatrist must base a diagnosis of, say, schizophrenia, solely on the symptoms manifested by his or her patient, without the help of either blood tests (as in malaria) or brain scans (as in stroke).

To do this, the psychiatrist must rely on clearly defined concepts and reliable diagnostic criteria. These are provided in classifications of mental disorders, and particularly in ICD-10 and

DSM-IV. The *ICD-10 Classification of Mental and Behavioural Disorders: clinical descriptions and diagnostic guidelines*, published in 1992, is chapter V of the *Tenth Revision of the International Classification of Diseases* (ICD-10). Unlike the other chapters, which simply list and code the names of diseases and disorders, chapter V also provides clinical descriptions and diagnostic criteria. These are based on scientific literature and international consultation and consensus, because ICD-10 is for use in all countries. The fourth revision of the *Diagnostic and Statistical Manual of Mental Disorders* (DSM-IV), first published in 1994 by the American Psychiatric Association, is an alternative but influential classification, and is broadly similar to the ICD-10 classification.

If the symptoms manifested by the patient tally with the diagnostic criteria for schizophrenia listed in ICD-10 or DSM-IV, then the psychiatrist is able to make a diagnosis of schizophrenia. However, he or she must also exclude psychiatric and medical conditions that can present like schizophrenia, for example, bipolar disorder, a head injury, or drug misuse. To do this, he or she must obtain a clear and detailed picture of the patient's symptoms and his personal and family history, usually over a protracted period of time. During this time, he or she may conduct a full physical examination, obtain blood and urine samples, and arrange for a non-invasive brain scan such as a computed tomography (CT) scan or a magnetic resonance imaging (MRI) scan. In some cases, he or she may also arrange for a second psychiatrist or other specialist (such as a neurologist or endocrinologist) to provide a second opinion. Only after confidently ruling out other psychiatric and medical conditions can the psychiatrist make a firm diagnosis of schizophrenia.

Coping with a diagnosis of mental disorder

A diagnosis of mental disorder such as schizophrenia or bipolar disorder can be difficult to accept, both for the person with the diagnosis and for his or her relatives. Like heart disease or diabetes, mental disorders can be serious and potentially debilitating illnesses. But unlike heart disease or diabetes, mental disorders are poorly understood and heavily stigmatised by the general public. This is in no small part due to the general public's lack of understanding of mental disorders, and to the sensationalist reporting in the media of violent acts committed by a very small number of people with psychotic disorders. The reality is that, while psychotic disorders such as schizophrenia and bipolar disorder are very common, they only rarely result in violent behaviour.

Owing to the stigma attached to a diagnosis of a psychotic disorder, some people may decide or be persuaded to consult a second or third psychiatrist – often at large expense – in the hope of having their diagnosis changed or reversed. Others may simply deny the diagnosis, and instead refer to their illness according to labels that they consider to be less stigmatising, such as 'depression' or 'anxiety disorder'. Some people may even prefer to tell others that they are in hospital because they have a brain tumour or because they are in a drug rehabilitation programme. Others, particularly if they are suffering from prominent delusions and hallucinations, may altogether deny that they are ill. After all, their delusions and hallucinations seem perfectly real to them, and they may even be positively brimming with energy and ideas. Making them see that they are ill can be a very tall task indeed.

In contrast, some people experience a great sense of relief at receiving a diagnosis of a psychotic disorder, because it enables them to get the help that they need, and so to make the fastest and most complete recovery possible. By accepting your psychiatrist's diagnosis, talking about it, reading about it, and seeking the help that you need, you are taking personal control over your illness and giving yourself the best chances of a long-term recovery. Remember that you are not alone, and that many people have once faced a similar situation. Talking to these people can provide you with much-needed information and support, and can help to alleviate any feelings of fear and isolation that you may have.

Unlike illnesses such as heart disease or diabetes, mental disorders such as schizophrenia and bipolar disorder tend to strike in the prime of life, when people are likely to be full of plans and dreams for the future. In some cases, they may feel under intense pressure to succeed and to be successful. As a result of being given a diagnosis of a serious mental disorder, they may feel that all their dreams have been shattered, and that they have betrayed those whom they hold most near and dear. Mixed feelings of loss, hopelessness, and guilt may give rise to, exacerbate, or prolong an episode of depression and, in some cases, even lead to thoughts of self-harm or suicide. In such cases, it is important to remember that increasing numbers of people who have been diagnosed with a serious mental disorder do make a durable recovery, and that many others nonetheless lead productive and fulfilling lives. Many people with a serious mental disorder, such as Winston Churchill (depression), Mark Twain (bipolar disorder), and John Nash (schizophrenia) have made unique and important contributions to society.

Finally, remember: you are not to blame for your illness, and you must not think that you have done anything to 'deserve it'. Do not let your parents blame themselves for your illness either. Just like anyone, people with a serious mental disorder can have good parents, bad parents, or absent parents. Far from being to blame, parents are often their child's most valuable source of structure and support, and their greatest hope for a permanent recovery. Serious mental disorders such as schizo-phrenia and bipolar disorder are common, and are in large part genetically determined. They are not anybody's fault.

Section 2

Master your mind through your mind

11 Building confidence and self-esteem

Low self-esteem can predispose you to developing a mental disorder, and developing a mental disorder can deliver a huge knock to your self-esteem. In some cases, low self-esteem is in itself a cardinal feature of mental disorder, for example, in depression or in borderline personality disorder. Thus, the relationship between low self-esteem and mental disorder is complex, and a person with a mental disorder is more likely than most to suffer from long-term low self-esteem. Self-esteem is also affected by physical ill-health, by negative life events such as losing your job or getting divorced, by poor relationships, and by a general sense of lack of control. Such a sense of lack of control is often particularly marked in people who are the victims of physical or sexual abuse, or of discrimination on the grounds of religion, culture, race, or sex.

Sometimes poor self-esteem can be deeply rooted and have its origins in traumatic childhood experiences such as prolonged separation from parent figures, neglect, or emotional, physical, or sexual abuse. If you think this is a particular problem for you, speak to your GP or to a member of your mental health-care team. Therapy or counselling may enable you to talk about such experiences and to try to come to terms with them. Unfortunately, therapy or counselling may be difficult to obtain, and may not be suitable for everyone.

People with long-term poor self-esteem generally see the world as a hostile place and themselves as its victim. As a result, they feel reluctant to express and assert themselves, miss out on experiences and opportunities, and feel helpless about changing things. All this merely lowers their self-esteem even further, and they end up getting caught in a downward spiral or vicious circle.

Thankfully, there are a number of simple things that anyone can do to boost his or her self-esteem and, hopefully, break out of this vicious circle. You may already be doing some of these things, and you certainly do not need to do them all. Just do those that you feel most comfortable with.

- Make three lists: one of your strengths, one of your achievements, and one of the things that you admire about yourself. Try to get a friend or relative to help you with these lists. Keep the lists in a safe place and read through them regularly.

- Think positively about yourself. Remind yourself that, despite your problems, you are a unique, special, and valuable person, and that you deserve to feel good about yourself. Identify and challenge any negative thoughts that you may have about yourself, such as 'I am a loser', 'I never do anything right', or 'No one really likes me'.

- Pay special attention to your personal hygiene: for example, style your hair, trim your nails, floss your teeth.

- Dress in clothes that make you feel good about yourself.

- Eat good food as part of a healthy, balanced diet. Make meal times a special time, even if you are eating alone. Turn off the TV or radio, set the table, and arrange your food so that it looks attractive on your plate.

- Exercise regularly: go out for a brisk walk every day, and take more vigorous exercise (exercise that makes you break into a sweat) three times a week.

- Ensure that you are getting enough sleep.

- Manage your stress levels. If possible, agree with a close friend or relative that you will take turns to massage each other on a regular basis.

- Make your living space clean, comfortable, and attractive. Display items that remind you of your achievements or of the special times and people in your life.

- Do more of the things that you enjoy doing. Do at least one thing that you enjoy every day, and remind yourself that you deserve it.

- Get involved in activities such as painting, music, poetry, and dance. Such artistic activities enable you to express yourself, acquire a sense of mastery, and interact positively with others. Find a class through your local adult education service or community centre.

- Set yourself a challenge that you can realistically achieve, and then go for it! For example, take up yoga, learn to sing, or cook for a small dinner party at your flat or house.

- Do some of the things that you have been putting off, such as clearing out the garden, washing the windows, or filing the paperwork.

- Do something nice for others. For example, strike up a conversation with the person at the till, visit a friend who is sick, or get involved with a local charity.

- Get others involved: tell your friends and relatives what you are going through and enlist their advice and support. Perhaps they have similar problems too, in which case you might be able to band up and form a support group.

- Try to spend more time with those you hold near and dear. At the same time, try to enlarge your social circle by making an effort to meet people.

- On the other hand, avoid people, places, and institutions that treat you badly or that make you feel bad about yourself. This could mean being more assertive. If assertiveness is a problem for you, ask your GP or another healthcare professional about assertiveness training.

12 Building relationships

Building relationships with other people is important for everyone, but particularly so for people who suffer from a mental disorder. Healthy, dependable relationships can provide you with practical and emotional support, and with the opportunity to discuss your thoughts and feelings freely and openly. This enables you not only to 'share the pain', but also to understand your thoughts and feelings better, and so to come to terms with them more readily. Spending time with others can pull you out of yourself, lift your mood, and boost your self-esteem. It can also provide you with a salutatory 'reality check', and help to correct any false beliefs that you may have.

The first rule of building relationships is simply to be authentic. Do not try to imagine what other people would like you to be like, and then play to the gallery. By being yourself from the start, you can quickly and instinctively gage whether you feel

Building relationships

comfortable with someone. This means that you can focus your attentions on nurturing each other and enjoying each other's company, rather than on playing empty mind games.

Of course no one is perfect, and you may need to make allowances for negative attributes. Sometimes a person's 'negative attributes' are not really negative attributes, but simply differences in opinions and interests. Try to respect these differences, to value them, and even to learn from them. And remember that, like authenticity, respect is usually reciprocated: the more you give, the more you receive in return.

Sometimes conflicts or tensions are inevitable. Conflicts are often silent and unspoken, so it is important to develop a sort of instinct for them. Once you have identified a conflict, bring it up at the soonest opportunity. Disclose your thoughts and feelings at a slow but steady rate. If you reveal too much too soon, you might end up feeling vulnerable or making the other person feel uncomfortable. Listen to the other person carefully, clarify his or her position, and make sure that there have been no misunderstandings. Do not assume that he or she knows what you want, and be very clear about what this is. However, do not simply expect him or her to cave in, and be prepared to negotiate and compromise. The best solution is usually the one that you both feel equally satisfied with, although in some cases it may be preferable or necessary for one of you to cave in. Remember that relationships should be mutually supportive, and that being supportive to another person can be very rewarding.

13
Managing stress

Stress can be an important problem in itself. However, it is a particular problem when it prevents a person from recovering from a mental disorder, or when it makes a person more vulnerable to a relapse in his or her mental disorder.

Stress is often related to 'life events', that is, important events such as losing a loved one, going through a divorce, losing a job, or falling ill. Life events can certainly be very stressful, but most of the stress that a person experiences on a daily basis comes from seemingly smaller 'background' stressors such as constant deadlines, tense relationships, painful memories (such as memories of physical or sexual abuse), isolation, discrimination, poor housing, or unpaid bills.

The amount of stress that a person can handle is largely related to his or her coping and thinking styles and level of social skills.

Managing stress

People with positive coping and thinking styles and good social skills are better able to diffuse stressful situations – for example, by doing something about them, by putting them in their proper context, or simply by talking about them and 'sharing the pain'.

The first step in dealing with stress is to be able to recognise its warning signs. Study Table 13.1 and write down on a piece of paper how you feel when you become stressed. Next make a list of situations in which you feel that way. For each situation on your list, think about one or more strategies that you can use to avoid it or make it less stressful. See Figure 13.1 for an example of such a list.

Table 13.1: Some of the symptoms of stress	
Emotional symptoms	Anxiety, fear, irritability, anger, resentment, loss of confidence, depression
Cognitive symptoms	Difficulty concentrating or making decisions, confusion, repetitive or circular thoughts
Physical symptoms	Dry mouth, tremor, sweatiness, racing heartbeat, chest tightness and difficulty breathing, muscle tension, headache, dizziness
Behavioural symptoms	Nervous habits such as nail biting or pacing, drinking more coffee and alcohol, eating too much or too little, sleeping poorly, acting brashly or unreasonably, losing your temper, being inconsiderate to others, neglecting your responsibilities

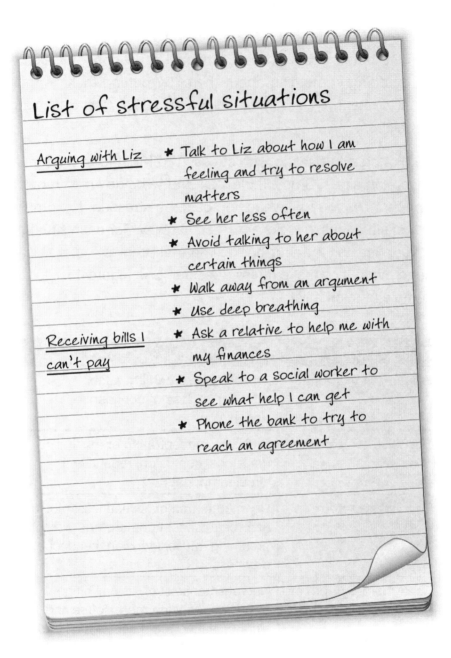

Figure 13.1 Make a list of situations which you find stressful and, for each situation on your list, think about one or more strategies for avoiding that situation or for making it less stressful.

Managing stress

There are also more general strategies that you can use for reducing stress. One common and effective strategy, called 'deep breathing', involves regulating your breathing:

- Breathe in through your nose and hold the air in for several seconds.

- Then purse your lips and gradually let the air out, making sure that you let out as much as you can.

- Continue doing this until you are feeling more relaxed.

A second strategy that is often used together with deep breathing involves relaxation exercises:

- Lying on your back, tighten the muscles in your toes for 10 seconds and then relax them completely.

- Do the same for your feet, ankles, and calves, gradually working your way up your body until you reach your head and neck.

Other general strategies that you can use for reducing stress include listening to classical music (for example, Bach or Chopin), taking a hot bath, reading a book or surfing the internet, calling up or meeting a friend, practising yoga or meditation, and playing sports.

Lifestyle changes can help both to reduce stress and to increase your ability to cope with stress. Lifestyle changes to consider include:

- Simplifying your life, even if this means doing less or doing only one thing at a time.

- Having a schedule and keeping to it.

- Getting enough sleep.

- Exercising regularly (for example, walking, swimming, doing yoga).

- Eating a balanced diet.

- Avoiding excessive caffeine or alcohol.

- Taking time out to do the things that you like doing.

- Connecting with others and sharing your problems with them.

- Changing your thinking style: having realistic expectations, reframing problems, expressing your feelings, maintaining a sense of humour.

Such lifestyle changes are good not only for managing stress, but also for your physical health and quality of life. Though individually small and simple, their cumulative effect can make a big difference to your prospects of making a durable recovery from mental disorder.

If coping with stress continues to be a problem, discuss this with your GP, psychiatrist, or key worker, and ask about relaxation training.

14 Managing anxiety

The first step in managing your anxiety is to learn as much as you can about it, as a thorough understanding of your anxiety can in itself reduce its frequency and intensity. It can be tempting to avoid the objects or situations that provoke your anxiety, but in the long run this is counterproductive. *When anxiety comes, accept it*. Do not try to escape from it. Simply wait and let it pass.

One effective method of coping with anxiety is to make a list of problems to overcome. Then break each problem down into a series of tasks, and rank the tasks in order of difficulty. For example, a person with arachnophobia (a phobia of spiders) may first think about spiders, then look at pictures of spiders, then look at real spiders from a safe distance, and so on. Attempt the easiest task first and keep on returning to it day after day, until you feel fairly comfortable with it. Give yourself as long as you need, then move on to the next task and do the same thing, and so on. Try to adopt a positive outlook: *although the symptoms of anxiety can be terrifying, they cannot harm you*.

If a given task is particularly anxiety-provoking, you can use relaxation techniques to manage your anxiety. These techniques can also be used more generally to reduce anxiety and stress. One common and effective relaxation technique, called 'deep breathing', involves regulating your breathing:

- Breathe in through your nose and hold the air in for several seconds.

- Then purse your lips and gradually let the air out, making sure that you let out as much as you can.

- Continue doing this until you are feeling more relaxed.

Another relaxation technique that is often used together with deep breathing involves relaxation exercises:

- Lying on your back, tighten the muscles in your toes for 10 seconds and then relax them completely.

- Do the same for your feet, ankles, and calves, and gradually work your way up your body until you reach your head and neck.

Other general strategies that you can use for relaxing include listening to classical music, taking a hot bath, reading a book or surfing the internet, calling up or meeting a friend, practising yoga or meditation, and playing sports. As you can see, there is no shortage of things you can do!

Managing anxiety

Simple lifestyle changes can also help to reduce your anxiety. These include:

- Structuring your day by having a schedule and keeping to it.

- Getting enough sleep.

- Exercising regularly (for example, walking, swimming, doing yoga).

- Eating a balanced diet.

- Avoiding excessive caffeine or alcohol.

- Taking time out to do the things that you like doing.

- Connecting with others and sharing your anxieties with them.

If you continue to suffer from severe anxiety despite following the advice given so far, you can get in touch with one of several voluntary organisations which, among others, operate telephone helplines and organise self-help groups. You can also speak to your GP who may suggest ways of helping you. For example, he or she may suggest referring you for a talking treatment, or starting you on antidepressant medication, which may be used in the treatment of both depressive disorders and anxiety disorders. If your anxiety is especially disabling, your GP may start you on a benzodiazepine sedative. Such sedatives are not in themselves a cure for anxiety, and are merely intended to provide you with short-term relief from your symptoms. Their long-term use should be avoided because they carry a high risk of dependence. 'Beta blockers' are also occasionally prescribed to control some of the symptoms of anxiety, such as the palpitations associated with a fast heart rate. They should be avoided in people with a history of heart problems or asthma.

Medication is usually most effective when it is combined with a talking treatment. Cognitive-behavioural therapy or CBT (see Module 39) is commonly used in the treatment of anxiety disorders. CBT for phobias may involve making a list of problems to overcome, and then breaking each problem down into a series of tasks that can be attempted in ascending order of difficulty. Relaxation techniques may also be taught so as to help you manage your anxiety and cope with each task more comfortably. CBT for panic disorder may also involve such graded exposure and relaxation training, but there is often also an added emphasis on modifying how you interpret changes in your body: for example, you may learn to interpret a fast heart rate in terms of the symptoms of anxiety, rather than 'catastrophically' in terms of having a heart attack. You may also be taught how to control your breathing so as to prevent hyperventilation, and thereby prevent some of the more alarming symptoms of anxiety. In CBT for post-traumatic stress disorder or PTSD, the emphasis is more on facing up to painful memories and images, and on learning to think about them in different ways.

15 Managing obsessions and compulsions

Antidepressant drugs (see Module 36) such as serotonin-selective reuptake inhibitors (SSRIs) and clomipramine are often prescribed for the treatment of obsessive-compulsive disorder, but obsessions and compulsions may also respond to cognitive-behavioural techniques, or to a combination of both antidepressant drugs and cognitive-behavioural techniques.

The most effective cognitive-behavioural technique for compulsions is to delay responding to your urges, and to distract yourself from the tension and anxiety that this provokes. Try to ignore your urges for longer and longer periods, so that you gradually get used to the discomfort that this gives rise to. By doing this, you basically short-circuit the vicious circle that dominates obsessive-compulsive thinking (Figure 15.1).

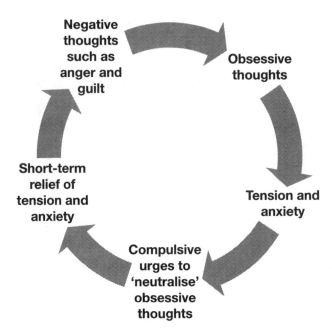

Figure 15.1 The vicious circle that takes hold in obsessive-compulsive disorder. Negative thoughts such as anger and guilt merely reinforce the original obsessional thoughts, setting up a vicious circle. You can break the vicious circle by ignoring your compulsive urges for longer and longer periods, and gradually getting used to the discomfort that this gives rise to.

Feeling tired or stressed (for example, because of a difficult relationship or a tight deadline) can aggravate your obsessive-compulsive symptoms, and ignoring your urges is going to be more challenging in these circumstances. Thus, whilst you can expect to make progress, you can also expect to have both good days and bad days. Do not feel discouraged by the bad days, but try to identify the stressor, and use the techniques for managing stress in Module 13 to deal with it.

Sometimes it can be helpful to devise an 'anxiety ladder', which involves ranking anxiety-provoking situations from 'least feared' to 'most feared' (Figure 15.2). Begin by exposing yourself to the first rung of your anxiety ladder and delay responding to your urges. Once you feel relatively comfortable with the first rung, move up to the next rung, and so on. Monitor your anxiety level as you delay responding to your urges, for example, by rating it on a scale of 0 to 10. After some time, your anxiety level should naturally begin to fall off. Sometimes it may seem impossible to prevent all your urges: if this is the case, try to gradually reduce the time that you spend carrying them out. For example, if your urge is to check the stove ten times, try to check it only five times.

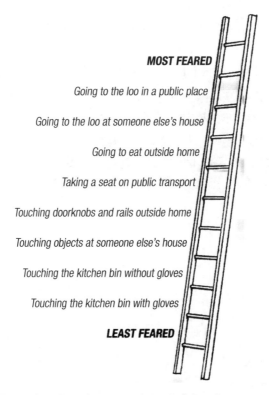

MOST FEARED

Going to the loo in a public place

Going to the loo at someone else's house

Going to eat outside home

Taking a seat on public transport

Touching doorknobs and rails outside home

Touching objects at someone else's house

Touching the kitchen bin without gloves

Touching the kitchen bin with gloves

LEAST FEARED

Figure 15.2 An example of an anxiety ladder for someone with an obsessional fear of germs and frequent and repetitive hand-washing.

Sometimes an obsessional thought or image may lead to a compulsion to have another thought or image so as to 'neutralise' it. A useful strategy for dealing with this is to stop fighting the original obsessional thought, and simply to accept it – however unnatural or difficult this may seem. Everyone has thoughts that can be unnatural, immoral, or violent; they are just thoughts, they do not make you a bad person. *If you try not to think about them, they only become more present in your mind*. To illustrate this point, try this now: try *not* to think about a pink elephant. Paradoxically, the only way not to think about a pink elephant is actually to think about it!

Finally, remember to feel positive above your achievements, however modest they may seem. Some people who resist their urges fall prey to negative thoughts. For example, they may feel guilty for putting their loved ones at risk by not checking the stove enough times. Such negative thoughts need to be identified and countered with 'reality testing'. An example of reality testing is to think to yourself, 'Most people do not check the stove 12 times.' See Module 16 for further advice on countering negative thoughts.

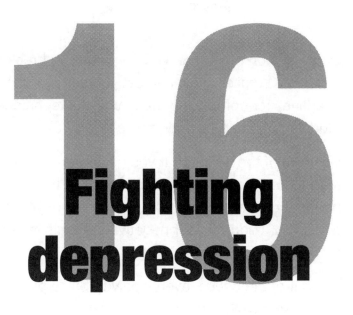

Fighting depression

There are a number of simple things that anyone can do to fight off depression. You may already be doing some of these things, and you certainly do not need to do them all. Just do those that you feel most comfortable with.

- Spend time with sympathetic friends and relatives, and talk to them about how you are feeling. If you do not feel comfortable speaking to friends and relatives, or are unable to, you can phone a helpline instead.

- Tell your friends and relatives that you need their time and help, and don't feel bad about letting them help you. They may well be able to offer you the company, patience, affection, understanding, encouragement, and support that you need.

- Don't take on more than you can manage: break large tasks into smaller ones, and set yourself realistic deadlines for completing them. Use the techniques in Module 13 to reduce your stress levels.

- Do more of the things that you usually enjoy doing: read a good book, go to the shops or to the cinema, visit friends – anything that gets you out of yourself and takes your mind off your negative thoughts is likely to make you feel better.

- Get out of the house, even if only to buy a pint of milk or to take a walk in the park.

- Take mild exercise, such as twenty minutes of brisk walking.

- Get sufficient amounts of sleep. Even a single good night's sleep can have a noticeable effect on your mood.

- Fight off your negative thoughts – perhaps the most important thing of all. Make a list of all the positive things about yourself (you may need help with this), keep it on you, and read it to yourself several times a day. However bad you may be feeling, remember that you have not always felt this way, and that you will not always feel this way. Have realistic expectations for yourself: improvements in mood are likely to be gradual rather than sudden, and there are going to be both good days and bad days.

- Avoid taking important decisions such as changing jobs or getting divorced while you are in the throes of depression. Thinking errors can lead you to make the wrong decisions. See the next module for more information on thinking errors.

- Ask your GP, psychiatrist, or key worker for advice.

Agree whom to call for advice and support should you feel overwhelmed by negative or suicidal thoughts. This may be a relative or friend, your key worker, or a helpline. Carry the appropriate telephone numbers on your person at all times, for example, in your wallet or handbag.

17 Thinking errors in depression

Thinking errors are irrational patterns of thinking that can both result in depression, and result from depression. The more depressed you feel, the more thinking errors affect you, and the more thinking errors affect you, the more depressed you feel. In order to break this vicious circle, you need to identify your thinking errors and to challenge them. Ask a trusted friend or relative for some help with this.

Some common thinking errors that result in and arise from depression include:

- Arbitrary inference, which involves drawing a conclusion in the absence of evidence. An example is, 'The whole world hates me.'

- Over-generalisation, which involves drawing a conclusion on the basis of very limited evidence. An example is, 'My nephew did not come to visit me. The whole world hates me.'

- Magnification and minimization, which involve either over- or under-estimating the importance of an event. An example is, 'Now that my cat is dead, I'll never have anything to look forward to.'

- Selective abstraction, which involves focusing on a single negative event or condition to the exclusion of other, more positive ones. For example, a person may be preoccupied by the fact that he or she is not currently in a relationship, but neglect the fact that he or she has a supportive family and a number of good friends.

- Dichotomous thinking, which involves 'all-or-nothing' thinking. A common example of dichotomous thinking in hospital in-patients with depression is, 'If he doesn't come to see me today, then he doesn't love me'. Another, more subtle, one is, 'If I'm not out of hospital by my daughter's birthday, she'll think that I don't love her.'

- Personalisation, which involves relating independent events to oneself. An example is, 'The nurse left her job because she was fed up with me'. (She more likely left because she got a promotion, or for family reasons).

- Catastrophic thinking, which involves exaggerating the consequences of an event or situation. An example is, 'The pain in my knee is getting worse. I'm probably going to end up in a wheelchair. Then I won't be able to go to work and pay the mortgage, so I'll lose my house and end up living on the street.'

18 Fighting thoughts of self-harm

Acts of self-harm are carried out for a variety of reasons, most commonly to express and relieve bottled-up anger or tension, feel more in control of a seemingly desperate life situation, punish oneself for being a 'bad person', or combat feelings of numbness and deadness and feel more 'connected' and alive. Acts of self-harm reflect very deep distress, and are most often used as a desperate and reluctant last resort – a method of surviving rather than of ending one's life, and sometimes also a method of attracting much-needed attention. For some people, the pain inflicted by self-harm is preferable to the numbness and emptiness that it replaces: it is something rather than nothing, and a salutatory reminder that one is still able to feel, that one is still alive. For others, the pain inflicted by self harm merely replaces a different kind of pain that they can neither understand nor control. Many people who self-harm feel that their behaviour is shameful, and such feelings may be reinforced by the stigma that they are unfairly made to feel.

Acts of self-harm are increasingly common in the UK, with approximately 170,000 cases presenting to hospitals each year. This is in itself a gross underestimate of the incidence of self-harm, as most cases are unlikely to present to hospital. The vast majority of cases that do present to hospital involve either a tablet overdose or self-cutting, although other forms of self-harm such as scratching or pulling out one's hair are also seen. Teenage girls are at the highest risk of self-harm, perhaps because older people have learned to deal better with their emotions, because they are better at hiding their self-harming activity, or because they self-harm only indirectly, for example, by misusing alcohol or drugs. The problems most frequently cited at the time of self-harm are problems with relationships, alcohol, employment, finances, housing, social isolation, bereavement, and physical health. Of the cases that present to hospital, about 25% report high suicidal intent, and about 40% are deemed to suffer from a major psychiatric disorder excluding personality disorder and alcohol or drug misuse. This means that the majority of people who self-harm are not deemed to be suffering from a major psychiatric disorder.

For some people, self-harm is a one-off response to a severe emotional crisis. For others it is a more long-term problem. Some people continue to self-harm because they continue to suffer from the same problems, or they may stop self-harming for a period – sometimes even several years – only to return to it at the next major emotional crisis. Of the cases that present to hospital, about 20–25% self-harm at least one more time in the following year.

If you are plagued by thoughts of self-harm, try to take your mind off them by using one of several coping strategies or distraction techniques. A useful coping strategy is to find someone you trust, such as a friend, relative, or teacher, and to share your feelings with him or her. If no one is available or there is no one you feel comfortable with, there are a number of emergency telephone lines that you can ring at any time. Engaging in creative activities such as writing, drawing, or playing a musical instrument can also take your mind off thoughts of harming yourself, and also help you to express your feelings and understand them better. Other coping strategies include reading a good book, listening to classical music, watching a comedy or nature programme, or even just cooking a meal or going out to the shops. Relaxation techniques like deep breathing (see Module 39) or yoga and meditation can also help. However, avoid alcohol and drugs as these can make your behaviour more impulsive, and significantly increase your likelihood of harming yourself. In some cases the urge to harm yourself may be so great that all you can do is to minimise the risks involved. Methods for doing this include holding ice cubes in your palm and attempting to crush them, fitting an elastic band around your wrist and flicking it, or plucking the hairs on your arms and legs.

If you have harmed yourself and are in pain or unable to control the bleeding, or if you have taken an overdose of any kind or size, call 999 immediately, or get a relative or friend to take you to Accident and Emergency as soon as possible. Going to Accident and Emergency not only enables you to get medical treatment, but also gives you an opportunity to spend time with someone and talk to him or her about your feelings.

Fighting thoughts of self-harm

Once things are more settled, consider getting yourself referred for a talking treatment such as counselling or cognitive-behavioural therapy (see Module 34). This can give you the opportunity to talk through your feelings in a safe and supportive environment, and to better understand why you sometimes feel the way you do. It can also help you to identify solutions to your problems, as well as alternative strategies for coping with them. Joining a local support group enables you to meet other people with similar problems to yours, that is, people who are likely to accept you and understand you, and with whom you may feel better able to share your feelings. However, beware of joining unmonitored online forums and chat groups, which are open to all and sundry, and which can sometimes leave you feeling even worse than before.

19 Fighting suicidal thoughts

Suicide was defined by the sociologist Emile Durkheim as applying to 'all cases of death resulting directly or indirectly from a positive or negative act of the victim himself, which he knows will produce this result'. In the UK there are around 5500 recorded suicides every year, and suicide is one of the leading causes of death among young adults. While deliberate self-harm is more common in women, completed suicide is three times more common in men. This may be because men are more likely to use violent and effective methods of suicide, or because men with suicidal thoughts find it more difficult to obtain and engage with the help and support that they need. According to the Office for National Statistics, the population group with the highest suicide rate is men aged from 25 to 44 years old, with a suicide rate of about 18 per 100,000 per year. One major problem with figures such as this one is that they reflect reported suicides, which in turn reflect verdicts reached in coroners' courts. *Actual* suicide rates may be considerably higher.

At the individual level, a person's risk of committing suicide can be increased by a number of demographic and social risk factors. Demographic risk factors for suicide include being male; being relatively young; and being single, widowed, or separated or divorced. Certain occupational groups such as veterinary surgeons, farmers, pharmacists, and doctors have been found to be at a higher risk of suicide. This is probably to do with their training and skills, and with their easy access to effective means of committing suicide, such as prescription-only drugs and firearms. Social risk factors for suicide include being unemployed, insecurely employed, or retired; having a poor level of social support as is often the case for the elderly, prisoners, immigrants, refugees, and the bereaved; and having been through a recent life crisis such as losing a close friend or relative or being the victim of physical or sexual abuse.

As well as demographic and social risk factors, a person's risk of committing suicide can also be increased by a number of clinical risk factors. The most important predictor of suicide is a previous act of deliberate self-harm, and a person's risk of completing suicide in the year following an act of deliberate self-harm is approximately 100 times greater than that of the average person. Conversely, up to half of all people who complete suicide have a history of deliberate self-harm. Suicidal behavior tends to cluster in families, so a family history of deliberate self-harm also increases a person's risk of suicide. This is perhaps because suicide is a learned behaviour or, more likely, because family members share a generic predisposition to psychiatric disorders that increase suicidal risk, such as schizophrenia, depression, bipolar disorder, personality disorders, and alcohol dependence. Some of these psychiatric disorders may, and often do, coexist, for example, personality disorder and alcohol dependence or schizophrenia and depression. People with a psychiatric disorder who are resistant to their prescribed medication or non-compliant with it are also at a higher risk of suicide, as are people experiencing certain specific symptoms such as delusions of persecution, delusions of control, delusions of jealousy, delusions of guilt, commanding second person auditory hallucinations (for example, a voice saying 'Take that knife and kill yourself'), and passivity which is the feeling that one's feelings, desires, and actions are under the control of an external agency. Physical illness can also increase the risk of suicide, and this is particularly the case for physical illnesses that are terminal, that involve chronic pain or disability, or that affect the brain. Examples of such physical illnesses include cancer, early-onset diabetes, stroke, epilepsy, multiple sclerosis, and AIDS.

If you are assailed by suicidal thoughts, the first thing to remember is that many people who have attempted suicide and survived ultimately feel relieved that they did not end their lives. At the time of attempting suicide they experienced intense feelings of despair and hopelessness, because it seemed to them that they had lost control over their lives, and that things could never get better. The only thing that they still had some control over was whether they lived or died, and so committing suicide seemed like the only option left. *This is never true.*

Fighting suicidal thoughts

Some of the thoughts that may accompany suicidal thoughts include:

- I want to escape my suffering.

- I have no other options.

- I am a horrible person and I do not deserve to live.

- I have betrayed my loved ones.

- My loved ones would be better off without me.

- I want my loved ones to know how bad I am feeling.

- I want my loved ones to know how bad they have made me feel.

Whatever thoughts you are having, and however bad you are feeling, remember that you have not always felt this way, and that you will not always feel this way.

The risk of committing suicide is highest in the combined presence of (1) suicidal thoughts, (2) the means to commit suicide, and (3) the opportunity to commit suicide. If you are prone to suicidal thoughts, ensure that the *means* to commit suicide have been removed. For example, give tablets and sharp objects to someone for safekeeping, or put them in a locked or otherwise inaccessible place. At the same time, ensure that the *opportunity* to commit suicide is lacking. The surest way of doing this is by remaining in close contact with one or more people, for example, by inviting them to stay with you. Share your thoughts and feelings with these people, and don't be reluctant to let them help you. If no one is available or no one seems suitable, there are a number of emergency telephone lines that you can ring at any time. You can even ring 999 for an ambulance or take yourself to an Accident and Emergency department. Do not use alcohol or drugs as these can make your behavior more impulsive, and significantly increase your likelihood of attempting suicide. In particular, do not drink or take drugs alone, or end up alone after drinking or taking drugs.

Make a list of all the positive things about yourself and a list of all the positive things about your life, including the things that have so far prevented you from committing suicide (you may need to get help with this). Keep the lists on you, and read them to yourself each time you are assailed by suicidal thoughts. On a separate sheet of paper, write a safety plan for the times when you feel like acting on your suicidal thoughts. Your safety plan could involve delaying any suicidal attempt by at least 48 hours, and then talking to someone about your thoughts and feelings as soon as possible. Discuss your safety plan with your GP, psychiatrist, or key worker and commit yourself to it. See Figure 19.1 for an example of a safety plan. Sometimes even a single good night's sleep can significantly alter your outlook, and it is important not to underestimate the importance that sleep can have. If you are having trouble sleeping, speak to a doctor.

Once things are a bit more settled, it is important that you address the cause or causes of your suicidal thoughts in as far as possible, for example, a mental disorder such as depression or alcohol dependence, a difficult life situation, or painful memories. Discuss this with your GP or another healthcare professional, who will help you to identify the most appropriate form of help available.

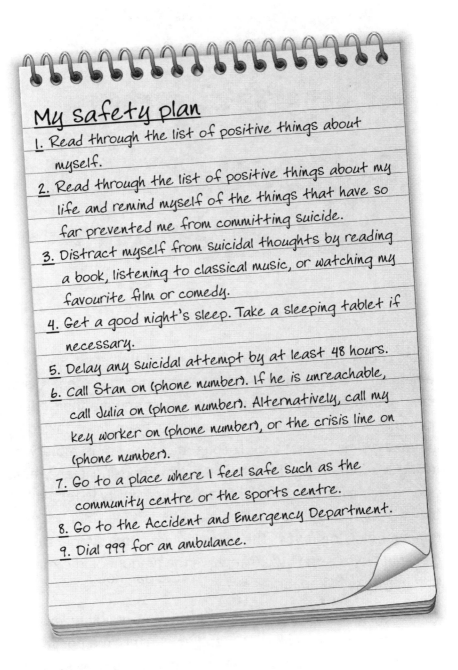

My safety plan
1. Read through the list of positive things about myself.
2. Read through the list of positive things about my life and remind myself of the things that have so far prevented me from committing suicide.
3. Distract myself from suicidal thoughts by reading a book, listening to classical music, or watching my favourite film or comedy.
4. Get a good night's sleep. Take a sleeping tablet if necessary.
5. Delay any suicidal attempt by at least 48 hours.
6. Call Stan on (phone number). If he is unreachable, call Julia on (phone number). Alternatively, call my key worker on (phone number), or the crisis line on (phone number).
7. Go to a place where I feel safe such as the community centre or the sports centre.
8. Go to the Accident and Emergency Department.
9. Dial 999 for an ambulance.

Figure 19.1 Example of a safety plan.

20 Improving concentration and memory

Many people with a mental disorder find that their ability to remember things is impaired by their mental disorder. This is most often because their mental disorder impairs their attention and concentration, which prevents them from taking in information in the first place. Thus, the problem is more with taking in information than with actually memorising it, and most people with a mental disorder find that their ability to remember things improves as they get better, and as their attention and concentration improves. The following are some simple strategies that anyone can use to improve the amount of information that they take in and remember:

- Pay attention. You cannot take in information unless you are paying attention, and you cannot memorise information unless you are taking it in. Get enough food and sleep, and avoid distractions such as a background radio or television.

Improving concentration and memory

- Involve as many senses as possible. For example, if you are sitting in a lecture, you will remember more of what is being said if you listen *and* scribble down a few notes. Or if you are reading a letter or an article, you will remember more of what is written if you read it aloud to yourself.

- Relate new information to what you already know. New information is much easier to remember if it can be contextualised. For example, if you are prescribed a new antidepressant drug, you can relate its side-effects to the side-effects of your old antidepressant drug. Or you might notice that both antidepressant drugs are from the same class of drugs, and thus that they have similar side-effects.

- Structure information. For example, if you need to remember what ingredients you need to cook a meal, think of them under the subheadings of starter, main course, and desert, and visualise how many ingredients there are under each sub-heading. Or if you need to remember a telephone number, think of it in terms of the five first digits, the middle three digits, and the last three digits.

- Use mnemonics, that is, tie information to visual images, sentences, acronyms, or rhymes. For example, you might remember that your hairdresser is called Sharon by picturing a Rose of Sharon or a sharon fruit. You might remember the order of the colours of the rainbow with the sentence, 'Richard of York got beaten in Versailles'. Or you might remember, as medical students do, the symptoms of varicose veins with the acronym 'AEIOU': aching, eczema, itching, oedema, and ulceration.

- Understand information. Try to understand more complex material before you try to remember it. If possible, summarise the material in your own words and write or type out your summary. Reorganise the material or your summary of the material so that it is easier to remember. By manipulating the information in this way, you are forcing yourself to think about it actively.

- Rehearse information. Review the information later on the same day or sleep over it and review it the following day. Thereafter, review it at regular, spaced intervals until you feel comfortable that you know it well enough.

- Exercise your mind. Mental challenge can help to create new wire connections in the brain, which makes it more effective and more resistant to memory disorders such as Alzheimer's disease. So develop a new hobby, read a novel, learn a foreign language, or practice yourself at the Times crossword.

- Develop a healthy lifestyle. Eat a healthy, balanced diet, take regular exercise, and avoid smoking. A healthy lifestyle increases the amount of blood and oxygen that is delivered to the brain, and reduces the risk of medical conditions that can lead to memory loss such as Alzheimer's disease, stroke, and diabetes. Exercise also increases your 'feel-good' endorphins, which improves your mood and prevents depression. As you might recall, depression results in impaired attention and concentration, and is also a risk factor for Alzheimer's disease.

- Get sufficient sleep. Sleep is necessary for memory consolidation, and feeling alert and refreshed improves your attention and concentration.

- See a doctor. Certain prescribed and over-the-counter drugs can impair your attention and concentration, and hence your memory. If you suspect that this is the case for you, see your GP or psychiatrist. You should also see your GP or psychiatrist if you begin having memory problems that affect your ability to get by on a day-to-day basis.

21 Coping with voices

Hallucinations can occur in schizophrenia, severe depression, mania, and some other mental disorders. Hallucinations can involve hearing, seeing, smelling, tasting, or feeling things that are not actually there. In most cases, they involve hearing voices. These voices can either speak directly *to* the person (second-person – 'you' – voices) or *about* him (third-person – 'he' – voices). Voices are often intensely distressing, particularly if they involve threats or abuse, or if they are loud or incessant. One might begin to experience something of this distress by turning on both the radio and television at the same time, both at full volume, and then trying to hold a normal conversation. While voices are usually distressing, they are not necessarily so. For example, some people with schizophrenia may get used to their voices and even begin to experience them as a source of comfort and reassurance. This is particularly likely

Coping with voices

if the voices are those of old acquaintances, dead ancestors, or 'guardian angels'.

Simple things that you can do to reduce or eliminate voices include:

- Find a trusted person to talk to about the voices. Do not be reluctant to accept help and support.

- Keep a diary of the voices to help you to identify and avoid situations in which they arise.

- Talk back to the voices: challenge them and ask them to go away. If you are out in public, you can avoid attracting attention to yourself by talking into a mobile phone.

- Drown out the voices by focusing your attention on an activity such as reading, gardening, singing, or listening to your favourite music.

- Think of the voices as what they are: nothing more than mere hallucinations.

- Reduce your levels of stress and anxiety (see Modules 13 and 14).

- Avoid drugs and alcohol (see Module 33).

- Take your medication as prescribed. If you are having problems taking your medication, speak to the doctor who prescribed it to you.

Coping with delusions and hallucinations (for carers)

Psychotic symptoms can be particularly distressing, both to the person experiencing them and to his or her carers. Carers often find themselves challenging the hallucinations and delusions, partly out of a desire to be helpful, and partly out of understandable feelings of fear and helplessness. Unfortunately this can be counterproductive, since it can alienate the person with a psychotic disorder from his or her carers at the very time that he or she needs them the most. Although this can be difficult, carers should remember that psychotic symptoms are as real to the person having them as they are unreal to everybody else.

So, a more helpful course of action for carers is to recognise that delusions and hallucinations are real and important to the person experiencing them, while making it clear that they themselves do not *personally* share in them. For example:

PERSON: An Archangel told me that I am the chosen one, and that my mission is to go forth and save mankind from sin.

CARER: Are you hearing him now?

PERSON: No, he's just stopped talking.

CARER: What else did he say?

PERSON: That to be successful I must confront the devil.

CARER: That sounds terrifying.

PERSON: I've never felt so frightened in all my life.

CARER: I can understand that you feel frightened, although I myself have never heard this archangel you speak about.

PERSON: You mean, you've never heard him?

CARER: No, not at all.

PERSON: What about the Devil? Have you heard him?

CARER: No, I haven't heard him either. Have you tried ignoring these voices?

PERSON: If I listen to my iPod then they don't seem so loud, and I don't feel so frightened.

CARER: What about when we talk together, like now?

PERSON: That's very helpful too.

23 Coping with high expressed emotion

Expressed emotion can be thought of as a specific type of stress. It refers to the amount of critical, hostile, or emotionally over-involved attitudes directed to a person with schizophrenia by his or relatives and carers. Such attitudes often originate in a misunderstanding that the person with schizophrenia is actually in control of his or her illness, and is 'choosing' to be ill. Alternatively, over-involvement may result from an unjustified sense of guilt about the illness, and a desire on the part of the relative or carer to 'share' the burden of the illness. A number of studies have demonstrated that high expressed emotion is an important risk factor for relapse in schizophrenia, and that it can increase the risk of relapse by *up to four times*. High expressed emotion from relatives and carers may lead a person with schizophrenia to feel trapped, helpless, or guilty, and the resultant stress may in itself provoke a relapse of the illness.

Coping with high expressed emotion

The relationship between high expressed emotion and schizo-phrenia is far from being a simple one: while high expressed emotion can precipitate a relapse of schizophrenia, it can also reflect legitimate feelings of anxiety and distress induced by illness in a loved one. It cannot be stressed enough that par-ents should not blame themselves for their son or daughter's illness. Instead, they should remind themselves that they are their child's most valuable source of structure and support, and his or her greatest hope for a permanent recovery.

If you feel that high expressed emotion is an issue for you or your family, speak to a member of your mental healthcare team about it. Expressed emotion is sometimes measured through a taped family interview known as the Camberwell Family Interview, or simply by interviewing the person with schizophrenia. Families with high expressed emotion may be offered educational ses-sions, stress management, or family therapy (see Module 34); these can all help to reduce expressed emotion, and can be important and integral parts of a person with schizophrenia's care plan. If relatives have a good understanding of the nature of schizophrenia, they are likely to be more understanding of the needs and demands of the person with schizophrenia and therefore less likely to contribute to high expressed emotion. Family therapy in particular requires a considerable investment of time and effort, but it may be particularly helpful if there are fundamental difficulties in the way that family members relate to one another. Family members should avoid nagging, criticis-ing, telling off, shouting, and arguing, and make sure to give the person with schizophrenia sufficient time and space to get better. This can be difficult to achieve, because it is often the instinct of family members to do as much as possible for their loved one, and because family members may have unrealistic expectations about the progress that their loved one ought to be making.

24 Coping with stigma

Facing other people can be one of the most difficult challenges for people with a mental disorder. The stigma attached to mental disorders, especially to schizophrenia and other psychotic disorders, arises from ignorance and the fear that is born out of it – a fear that is all too often reinforced by the misrepresentation of people with mental disorders in the media.

As a group people with a mental disorder are not unpredictable or dangerous; they are not lazy or 'moral failures'; and getting better is not simply a matter of them 'pulling themselves together'. Severe forms of mental disorder have a strong biological basis and are certainly not 'all in the mind'.

For people with a mental disorder, stigma can create a vicious circle of alienation and discrimination that hinders progress to recovery by promoting anxiety, depression, alcohol and drug misuse, social isolation, unemployment, homelessness, and institutionalisation. Many people with a mental disorder report that the stigma that they are made to feel can be even more distressing than their symptoms; in some cases they fear this stigma to such an extent that they are unable to accept that they are ill, and so do not seek out the help that they need.

For all this, mental disorders are very common. According to a World Health Organization (WHO) report, one in four people in the world will suffer from a mental health problem at some point in their life. In the UK mental health accounts for up to one third of all general practice consultations, and every year the National Health Service (NHS) spends more money on mental healthcare than on any other area of healthcare, including cardiovascular disease, cancer, and even primary care.

Furthermore, some of the most creative and successful people in society suffer or suffered from a mental disorder. Highly creative people who suffered from depression include Charles Baudelaire, Winston Churchill, Hart Crane, Charles Dickens, William Faulkner, Michel Foucault, Graham Greene, William James, Abraham Lincoln, John Stuart Mill, Isaac Newton, Friedrich Nietzsche, Rainer Maria Rilke, Arthur Schopenhauer, Leo Tolstoy, Evelyn Waugh, and Tennessee Williams.

Highly creative people who suffered from bipolar disorder include the authors Hans Christian Andersen, Honoré de Balzac, F. Scott Fitzgerald, Ernest Hemingway, Victor Hugo, Edgar Allan Poe, Mary Shelley, Mark Twain, and Virginia Woolf; the poets William Blake, Emily Dickinson, TS Eliot, John Keats, Robert Lowell, Sylvia Plath, Alfred Lord Tennyson, and Walt Whitman; and the composers Ludwig van Beethoven, Hector

Coping with stigma

Berlioz, George Frederic Handel, Gustav Mahler, Sergei Rachmaninoff, Robert Schumann, and Peter Tchaikovsky.

Highly creative people who suffered from schizophrenia include Syd Barrett (1946–2006), the early driving force behind the rock band Pink Floyd; John Nash (born 1928), the father of 'game theory' and Nobel Prize winner; and Vaclav Nijinsky (1889–1950), the legendary choreographer and dancer. Many more highly creative people, while not suffering from schizophrenia themselves, have or have had close relatives who do. This was, for example, the case for the physicist Albert Einstein (his son had schizophrenia), the philosopher Bertrand Russell (also his son), and the novelist James Joyce (his daughter).

Despite all this, many people with a mental disorder feel unable to talk about their difficulties for fear of the hurt and shame of being stigmatised. Being open about your illness may be a risk, but it also enables you to talk about your feelings, and to gain the support that you need. Learn as much as you can about your illness so that you yourself can correct any false beliefs that people may hold about it. Try to educate friends and relatives about your illness and the issues surrounding it. If people use derogatory terms such as 'maniac' or 'psycho', remind them that their behaviour is unacceptable. If you feel that you are being unfairly treated as a customer or service user, make a complaint. You can even take a public stance against discrimination – for example, by speaking at events, or writing about your experiences on a blog or in a local newspaper or magazine. Joining a local support group enables you to meet other people with similar problems to the ones that you are having, and so to escape stigma (even if only temporarily). You can also use support groups to share your experiences and learn from and support one another.

Relatives, friends, and carers should analyse their attitudes and behaviours, and ensure that they are not involuntarily contributing to the stigma felt by the person whom they are caring for. Attitudes and behaviours that contribute to stigma are often subtle, and may, for example, involve talking to people with a mental disorder as if they are children or as if they are hard of hearing, talking about them as if they are not in the room, and failing to grant them sufficient autonomy and responsibility. A simple rule of thumb for relatives, friends, and carers is to behave towards the person whom they are caring for as they would towards any other person: naturally, simply, and with due respect and courtesy. Carers should try to be a 'refuge' or 'comfort zone' for the person whom they are caring for, offering him or her practical and emotional support, but also the space and time to be quiet and alone. Deep questioning, argument, and the venting of intense negative emotions may overwhelm a person with a mental disorder, and need to be avoided.

25 Preventing relapses

Relapses can have devastating consequences for people with mental disorders such as schizophrenia, bipolar disorder, depression, or an anxiety disorder. After every relapse, it may become increasingly difficult to regain control over the symptoms. For this reason, it is especially important for people with a mental disorder to do all that is possible to reduce the risk of a relapse.

Scientific research suggests that, in many cases, long-term treatment with medication can substantially reduce the risk of relapse. If you are reluctant to take your medication because the schedule is too complicated or because you are suffering from side-effects that you find unacceptable, speak to your GP or psychiatrist about this. Your GP or psychiatrist may be able to simplify the schedule, decrease the dose, or change you to another medication that suits you better. *Do not simply stop taking your medication*. Unfortunately, taking your medication at the dose prescribed by your GP or psychiatrist is often the single most important thing that you can do to prevent a relapse.

People with a mental disorder and their relatives, friends, and carers should learn to recognise the early signs and symptoms of a relapse. These signs and symptoms may differ from one person to another and from one mental disorder to another, but common ones include:

- Suffering changes in mood.

- Losing your sense of humour.

- Becoming tense, irritable, or agitated.

- Finding it difficult to concentrate.

- Retreating from social situations and neglecting outside activities and social relationships.

- Saying or doing irrational or inappropriate things.

- Developing ideas that other people find unusual, strange, or unbelievable.

- Neglecting your personal care.

- Neglecting to take your medication.

- Dressing in unusual clothes or unusual combinations of clothes.

- Sleeping excessively or hardly at all.

- Eating excessively or hardly at all.

- Becoming increasingly suspicious or hostile.

- Becoming especially sensitive to noise or light.

- Hearing voices or seeing things that other people cannot see or hear.

If you notice or suspect any of these signs and symptoms in yourself, contact your GP, psychiatrist, or key worker as soon as possible for support and advice, as this may help to avert a full-scale relapse. Before problems arise, it is a good idea to have an action plan in place, and to have discussed this action plan with your GP, psychiatrist, or key worker. You can also keep a diary to help you identify the signs and symptoms of a possible relapse. Remember that a relapse may impair your thinking, and so prevent you from recognising those signs and symptoms. You may therefore need to rely on family, friends, and carers, and to trust in their judgement.

Try to identify any factors that may have caused or contributed to your signs and symptoms, because addressing these factors may help you to avert a full-scale relapse. Some of the most important factors that may cause or contribute to a relapse are listed in Table 25.1 and discussed more fully in other sections of this book. Minimising them can help you to prevent relapses, and so significantly improve your chances of making a durable recovery.

Table 25.1: Some of the most important factors that may cause or contribute to a relapse
• Poor understanding of your mental disorder in general, and of the symptoms of a relapse in particular • Non-compliance with medication or decreased dose of medication • Drug and alcohol misuse • Lack of sleep or irregular pattern of sleep • Stress • Lack of social relationships and support • Felt stigma • Poor physical health

26 Aristotle on human flourishing

In his Nicomachean Ethics, the Greek philosopher Aristotle (d. 322 BC) tries to discover what is 'the supreme good for man', that is, what is the best way to lead our life and to give it meaning. For Aristotle, a thing is best understood by looking at its end, purpose, or goal. For example, the purpose of a knife is to cut, and it is by seeing this that one best understands what a knife is; the goal of medicine is good health, and it is by seeing this that one best understands what medicine is.

If one does this for some time, it soon becomes clear that some goals are subordinate to other goals, which are themselves subordinate to yet other goals. For example, a medical student's goal may be to qualify as a doctor, but this goal is subordinate to his goal to heal the sick, which is itself subordinate to his goal to make a living by doing something useful. This could go on and on, but unless the medical student has a goal that is an end-in-itself, nothing that he does is actually worth doing.

What, asks Aristotle, is this goal that is an end-in-itself? The supreme Good, says Aristotle, is happiness:

> And of this nature Happiness is mostly thought
> to be, for this we choose always for its own sake,
> and never with a view to anything further: whereas
> honour, pleasure, intellect, in fact every excellence
> we choose for their own sakes, it is true, but
> we choose them also with a view to happiness,
> conceiving that through their instrumentality we
> shall be happy: but no man chooses happiness
> with a view to them, nor in fact with a view to any
> other thing whatsoever.

But what is happiness? For Aristotle, it by understanding the distinctive function of a thing that one can understand its essence. Thus, one cannot understand what it is to be a gardener unless one can understand that the distinctive function of a gardener is 'to tend to a garden with a certain degree of skill'. Whereas human beings need nourishment like plants, and have sentience like animals, their distinctive function, says Aristotle, is their unique capacity to reason. Thus the supreme Good, or happiness, is to lead a life that enables us to use and to develop our reason, and that is in accordance with rational principles. In contrast to amusement or pleasure which can also be enjoyed by animals, happiness is not a state but an activity, and it is profound and enduring.

Aristotle on human flourishing

Aristotle acknowledges that our good or bad fortune can play a part in determining our happiness; for example, he acknowledges that happiness can be affected by such factors as our material circumstances, our place in society, and even our looks. Yet he maintains that by living our life to the full according to our essential nature as rational beings, we are bound to become happy regardless. For this reason, happiness is more a question of behaviour and of habit – of 'virtue' – than of luck; a person who cultivates such behaviours and habits is able to bear his misfortunes with equanimity, and thus can never be said to be truly unhappy.

Section 3

Master your mind through your body

27 Monitoring your physical health

Compared with other groups of people, people with a mental disorder are more likely to eat poorly, lack exercise, smoke, and use alcohol and drugs. For these reasons they are more likely to suffer from obesity; diabetes; cardiovascular problems such as high blood pressure, heart attack, and stroke; and respiratory problems such as chronic bronchitis and emphysema. Some of the possible side-effects of medication (for example, antipsychotic medication, lithium, or valproate) can directly or indirectly contribute to problems such as obesity and diabetes, making the care of your physical health all the more important.

Physical health problems do not affect everyone with a mental disorder, but it is important that you have your physical health monitored so that any eventual problems can be detected early on. Your GP is normally able to carry out a physical check once every year. This usually involves weighing you, taking your pulse rate and blood pressure, and carrying out a blood or urine test. A physical check is also a good opportunity to discuss your symptoms and medication, and to obtain advice on maintaining a healthy lifestyle.

Maintaining a healthy lifestyle is the key to good physical health, and basically involves eating healthily (Module 28), taking exercise (Module 29), sleeping well (Module 30), and – if necessary – quitting smoking (Module 31) and quitting alcohol and drugs (Module 32).

28
Eating healthily

There are two separate factors to consider about your diet:

- Whether you are eating the right amount to keep your weight in the desirable range for health.

- Whether you are eating a healthy balanced diet.

Consult a height–weight chart (Figure 29.1) to check whether you are the right weight for your height.

If you are underweight for your height, this may be a cause for concern, and you should try to put on weight through eating sufficient quantities of a healthy, balanced diet. If this fails or if you are significantly underweight, consult your GP for further advice.

If you are overweight for your height, try to cut down on the amount that you are eating, especially on foods that are high

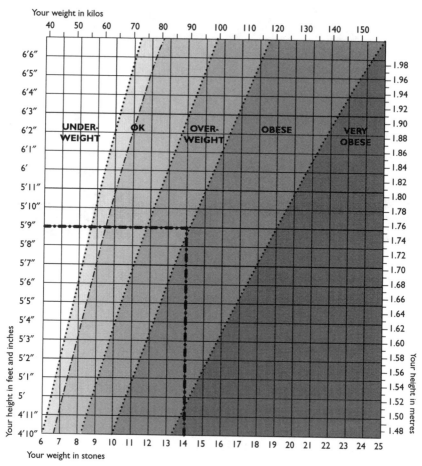

Figure 29.1 Height–weight chart.

in sugar or saturated and hydrogenated fats, and try to take more exercise (see the next Module). If you are obese or very obese for your height, you are at a high risk of physical health problems such as diabetes, high blood pressure, heart problems, and stroke. It is particularly important that you try to lose weight, but be realistic about what you can achieve: rather than go on to a 'crash diet' that is bound to end in failure, aim to lose small amounts of weight steadily over a longer period of time.

Cut back on foods that are high in sugar or saturated and hydrogenated fats such as fried foods, meat products, hard cheese, cream, and butter. Eat three meals a day, but avoid snacking in between meals, especially on 'comfort' foods such as chocolate, cakes, biscuits, and crisps. If you do feel like snacking, prefer a piece of fruit such as an apple, pear, or banana. If you have had problems trying to lose weight in the past, consult your GP or a dietician for further advice.

If your weight is OK for your height, then you are eating about the right amount to keep your weight in the desirable range for health. This does not, however, mean that you are necessarily eating a healthy balanced diet.

What is a healthy balanced diet?

A healthy balanced diet:

- Is based on starchy foods such as wholegrain bread, potatoes, pasta, and rice.
- Contains a lot of fruit and vegetables (five portions a day).
- Contains some protein-rich foods such as fish, poultry, meat, eggs, and pulses.
- Is low in fat, sugar, and salt.

How do I maintain a healthy balanced diet?

Here are eight tips for eating well from eatwell, the UK Food Standards Agency consumer advice and information website (www.eatwell.gov.uk):

1. Base your meals on starchy foods.

2. Eat lots of fruit and vegetables.

3. Eat more fish.

4. Cut down on saturated fat and sugar.

5. Try to eat less salt – no more than 6 grams a day.

6. Get active and try to be a healthy weight.

7. Drink plenty of water.

8. Don't skip breakfast.

If you are eating a healthy balanced diet, you are most probably getting all the vitamins and minerals that your body needs, and you do not need to take any dietary supplements.

29
Taking exercise

Regular exercise is an important part of looking after both your physical health and your mental health.

With regard to your physical health, exercise helps you to become and to remain slim. It also decreases your blood pressure, increases your physical strength and endurance, and improves your posture and flexibility. Exercise also improves the quality of your sleep, although it should not be taken just before bed time because its short-term alerting effects may prevent you from falling asleep.

With regard to your mental health, exercise helps to decrease stress, improve thinking and motivation, boost self esteem, and lift mood by causing the body to release greater amounts of chemical messengers called endorphins. Exercise can also give you something to look forward to, and something to help structure your day.

Exercise does not have to be difficult or intensive, and 30 minutes of moderate activity a day is all that is needed to improve your fitness. You could do some gardening, walk to the shops, cycle, exercise at a gym or swimming pool, or play a team sport such as basketball or football. In fact, there are so many possibilities to choose from that you are bound to find one that you enjoy doing. By getting you out of the house and 'out of yourself', exercise can remove you from emotional conflict, distract you from your symptoms, and increase the number and frequency of your social interactions. This in itself can have a major positive effect on your mental health.

The various benefits of taking exercise are summarised in Table 29.1.

Table 29.1: Some of the possible benefits of taking exercise
• Weight loss
• Decreased blood pressure
• Increased physical strength and endurance
• Improved posture and flexibility
• Better sleep
• Better appetite
• Decreased stress
• Improved thinking and motivation
• Bolstered self-esteem
• Improved mood
• Removal from emotional conflict
• Distraction from symptoms of mental disorder
• Increased social interactions

30
Sleeping well

Insomnia – difficulty in falling asleep or staying asleep – affects 30 per cent of people, but is even more common in people with a mental illness in whom it can be a direct effect of the illness. Insomnia is usually a problem if it occurs on most nights and causes distress or daytime effects such as fatigue, poor concentration, poor memory, and irritability. These symptoms may not only delay your recovery, but may also predispose you to accidents, to depression and anxiety, and to medical disorders such as infections, high blood pressure, obesity, and diabetes. Insomnia can also be caused or aggravated by poor sleep habits, depression, anxiety, stress, physical problems such as pain or shortness of breath, certain medications, and alcohol or drug use (see Table 30.1). Short-term insomnia specifically is often caused by a stressful life event, a poor sleep environment, or an irregular routine.

> ### Table 30.1: Some of the commoner causes of insomnia
>
> - Poor sleep habits
> - Psychiatric disorders
>   - Depressive disorder
>   - Mania and bipolar affective disorder
>   - Anxiety disorders
>   - Schizophrenia
>   - Post-traumatic stress disorder
>   - Chronic fatigue syndrome
> - Medical disorders
>   - Restless leg syndrome (thrashing about during sleep)
>   - Sleep apnoea (snoring with pauses in breathing)
>   - Chronic pain
>   - Chronic obstructive pulmonary disease
>   - Chronic renal failure
>   - Neurological disorders such as Parkinson's disease
>   - Headaches
>   - Fibromyalgia
> - Other
>   - Alcohol and drug misuse
>   - Side effects of medication such as antipsychotic or antidepressant medication
>   - Shift working
> - Caring for young children

If you are suffering from insomnia, there are a number of simple measures that you can take to resolve or at least lessen the problem:

- Have a strict routine involving regular and adequate sleeping times (most adults need about seven or eight hours of sleep every night). Allocate a time for sleeping, for example, 11pm to 7am, and do not use this time for any other activities. Avoid daytime naps, or make them short and regular. If you have a bad night, avoid 'sleeping in' because this makes it more difficult to fall asleep the following night.

- Have a relaxing bedtime routine that enables you to relax and 'wind down' before bedtime. This may involve doing breathing exercises or meditation or simply reading a book, listening to music, or watching TV.

- Many people find it helpful to have a hot drink: if this is the case for you, prefer a herbal or malted or chocolate drink to stimulant drinks such as tea or coffee.

- Sleep in a familiar, dark, and quiet room that is adequately ventilated and neither too hot nor too cold. Try to use this room for sleeping only, so that you come to associate it with sleeping.

- If you can't sleep, don't become anxious and try to force yourself to sleep. The more anxious you become, the less likely you are to fall asleep, and this is only likely to make you more anxious! Instead, get up and do something relaxing and enjoyable for about half an hour, and then try again.

- Take regular exercise during the daytime, but do not exercise in the evening or just before bedtime because the short-term alerting effects of exercise may prevent you from falling asleep.

- Try to reduce your overall levels of stress by implementing some of the lifestyle changed suggested in Module 13.

- Eat an adequate evening meal containing a good balance of complex carbohydrates and protein. Eating too much can make it difficult to fall asleep; eating too little can disturb your sleep and decrease its quality.

- Avoid alcohol, caffeine, and tobacco, particularly in the evening. Also avoid stimulant drugs such as cocaine, amphetamines, and ecstasy. Alcohol may make you fall asleep more easily, but it decreases the quality of your sleep.

If insomnia persists despite these measures, seek advice from your GP or psychiatrist. In some cases, insomnia may have a clear and definite cause that needs to be addressed in itself – for example, a physical problem or a side-effect of medication. Behavioural interventions such as sleep restriction therapy or cognitive-behavioural therapy can be helpful in some cases, and are preferable to sleeping tablets in the long-term. Sleeping tablets can be effective in the short-term, but are best avoided in the longer term because of their side-effects and their high potential for tolerance (meaning that you need progressively higher doses to achieve the same effect) and dependence. Sleeping remedies that are available without a prescription often contain an antihistamine that can leave you feeling drowsy the following morning. If you decide to use such remedies, it is important that you do not drive or operate heavy machinery the next day. Herbal alternatives are usually based on the herb valerian, a hardy perennial flowering plant with heads of sweetly scented pink or white flowers. If you are thinking about using a herbal remedy, speak to your GP or psychiatrist first, particularly if you have a medical condition or allergy, if you are already on medication, or if you are pregnant or breast-feeding.

Sleeping well

For people with bipolar disorder, loss of sleep or irregular sleep patterns can trigger a manic episode. Even going to bed unusually late – for example, after having to meet an important deadline or after a big night out – can be sufficient to trigger a manic episode. For this reason, people with bipolar disorder who are students at university, work long hours, or work shifts are at an especial risk of developing a manic episode. People with bipolar disorder may also develop a manic episode after travelling across several time zones and needing to readjust their circadian rhythms and sleep patterns. If a person's mood becomes even slightly abnormally elevated, he or she may be unable to sleep. As sleep is lost, his or her mood is likely to become even more abnormally elevated. As you can see, a vicious circle quickly takes hold. For the person with bipolar disorder, it is all-important to recognise this vicious circle early and to try to cut it short.

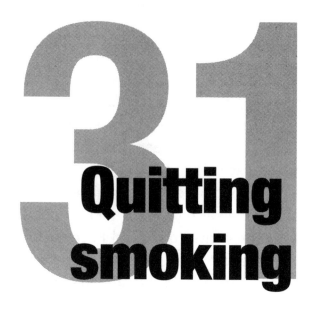

31 Quitting smoking

People with a mental disorder, particular a psychotic disorder such as schizophrenia, are much more likely to take up smoking than the average person. They are also more likely to smoke heavily, with dire consequences for their physical health, quality of life, and life expectancy. Indeed, cardiovascular and respiratory diseases that are both caused and aggravated by smoking are among some of the most common causes of death in people with schizophrenia. Smoking also results in a decrease in blood levels of antipsychotic medication, such that smokers require higher doses of antipsychotic medication than non-smokers to achieve the same therapeutic effect. And assuming that a pack of 20 cigarettes costs an average of £5.50, someone smoking 40 cigarettes a day spends (£5.50 × 2) × 365 = £4,015 on cigarettes each year. Although roll up cigarettes are cheaper than filter cigarettes, they can also be more damaging to physical health.

Many people with a psychotic disorder who smoke started smoking before they became ill, suggesting either that smoking predisposes to psychotic disorders or, more likely, that the genetic or environmental factors that predispose to psychotic disorders also predispose to nicotine addiction. An alternative explanation for the high rates of smoking in people with psychotic disorders is that their illness makes them more likely to smoke because they feel that smoking alleviates their symptoms or helps them to relax.

A commonly held perception is that people with a psychotic disorder are unlikely to give up smoking and that it is unfair or even inhumane to try to deprive them of one of their principal pastimes and pleasures. The truth is that many people with a psychotic disorder are highly motivated to stop smoking and are in need of all the help that they can get to fight what is often a severe nicotine addiction. Help can take the form of smoking cessation groups, behavioural therapy, nicotine replacement (in the form of patches or lozenges, for example), and alternative therapies such as acupuncture and hypnosis. Success rates vary greatly from one person to another, but it is important to keep on persisting.

If you want to stop smoking, talk to your GP, psychiatrist, or key worker. Further information and support is also available from

www.netdoctor.co.uk/smoking/index.shtml

How can I begin to stop smoking?

Make a list of the pros and cons of smoking. See Figure 31.1 for an example of such a list.

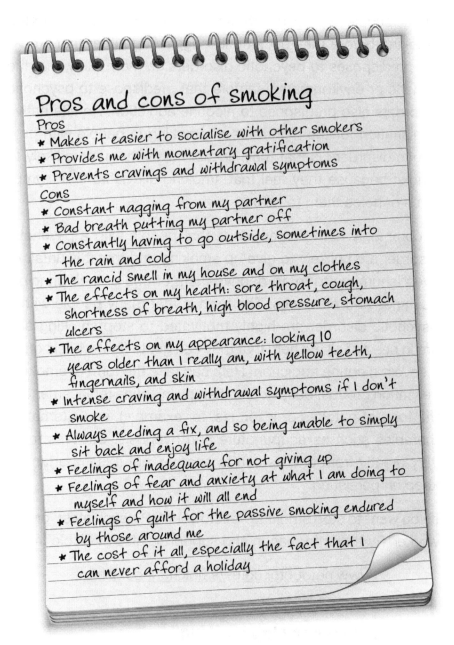

Figure 31.1 One person's list of the pros and cons of smoking.

Quitting smoking

Keep your list on you and use it to motivate yourself to quit. Choose a date on which you want to quit and stick to it. Between now and that date keep a log of your smoking habits: record the times at which you 'light up', where you are, what you are doing, and how you are feeling. Use this log to get a better understanding of your pattern of smoking. Once your chosen date arrives, make a clean break by throwing out all cigarettes and removing all ashtrays, lighters, and matches. You are likely to experience intense cravings and withdrawal symptoms such as irritability, difficulty concentrating, tiredness, headache, increased appetite, and insomnia. Nicotine replacement can help to relieve these cravings and withdrawal symptoms, so ask your GP or psychiatrist about them. Cravings rarely last for more than a couple of minutes at a time, and diversion techniques such as chewing gum, brushing your teeth, or doing a crossword puzzle may take your mind off them until they pass. If these diversion techniques fail, call a friend or relative who knows what you are going through, and who has agreed to offer you help and support. Alternatively, read your list of pros and cons and use it to motivate yourself. Cravings are often triggered by certain places, activities, and emotions that you have come to associate with lighting up. Use the log of your smoking habits to identify these places, activities, and emotions, and try to think of alternative coping strategies to smoking.

Remember: cravings and withdrawal symptoms do not last for ever, and in a matter of only days quitting will have become a much easier task! Don't be too harsh on yourself if you give in to temptation: put it behind you and keep on trying your best.

Staying off alcohol and drugs

People with a mental disorder who drink heavily or use illicit drugs are likely to delay their recovery, and are likely to suffer more frequent and more severe relapses. Those with symptoms of anxiety, depression, or psychosis may turn to alcohol or illicit drugs such as cannabis, amphetamines, and heroin to obtain relief from their symptoms. Alcohol and drugs may temporarily blunt or mask symptoms, but in the long run they are likely to lead to more severe symptoms and to more frequent and more severe relapses. A vicious circle takes hold whereby the more people use alcohol and illicit drugs to mask their symptoms, the worse their symptoms become; and the worse their symptoms become, the more they need to use alcohol and illicit drugs to mask them. Alcohol and drugs may also delay people with a mental disorder from getting the help that they need, including – in some cases – getting an all-important prescription for medication.

Staying off alcohol and drugs

Apart from this, possible consequences of alcohol and drug use include:

- Increased psychotic symptoms.

- Reduced response to medication.

- Reduced compliance with medication.

- Medical complications such as high blood pressure, heart attack, stroke, stomach ulcers, and liver disease.

- Complications of intravenous drug use such as hepatitis, HIV infection, and venous thrombosis.

- Death by accidental overdose.

- Family and marital difficulties.

- Motoring offences.

- Accidents.

- Financial hardship.

- Criminal activity and its consequences.

Should you need it, simple advice and support is readily available from your GP or Community Mental Health Team. You may find it useful to ask a healthcare professional to help you to devise a goal-oriented care and treatment plan that is tailored to your needs. Tasks in this care and treatment plan could in the first instance include, for example, keeping your appointments, keeping a diary of alcohol or drug use, and taking your prescribed medication. Relatives and friends can play an important role in supporting and monitoring progress, and they should, if possible, be included in the care and treatment plan. They should try to adopt an open and non-judgemental approach, in an attempt to bolster the self-esteem of the person they are caring for and to make him or her feel in greater control of the problem.

Alcohol or drug use is often promoted by stressful situations, so learning techniques for managing stress and anxiety, such as deep breathing and progressive muscle relaxation, can be particularly helpful, as can be learning and role-playing specific social skills which can then be deployed in stressful and high-risk situations. Such social skills may for example involve going into a pub and ordering a non-alcoholic drink, or saying 'no' to a drug dealer.

If you find yourself in a stressful situation and are about to give in to temptation, don't! Call a relative or friend, talk through the situation, and get the support and encouragement that you need to pull through. Some people with a mental disorder also find support and encouragement in local support groups, or in more structured so-called '12-step programmes' such as Alcoholics Anonymous or Narcotics Anonymous. Ask your GP, psychiatrist, or key worker if such groups are suitable for you.

Alcoholics Anonymous

Founded in 1935 in Ohio, Alcoholics Anonymous is a spiritually oriented community of alcoholics whose aim is to stay sober and, through shared experience and understanding, to help other alcoholics to do the same, 'one day at a time', by avoiding that first drink. The essence of the programme involves a 'spiritual awakening' that is achieved by 'working the steps', usually with the guidance of a more experienced member or 'sponsor'. Members initially attend daily meetings in which they share their experiences of alcoholism and recovery and engage in prayer and meditation. A prayer that is usually recited at every meeting is the Serenity Prayer, the short version of which goes:

God grant me the serenity to accept the things I
  cannot change,
Courage to change the things I can,
And the wisdom to know the difference.

Section 4

Psychological and physical treatments

Psychological or 'talking' treatments

Although drug treatments are the most readily available treatment option for mental disorders such as anxiety and depression, psychological or 'talking' treatments can in many cases be more effective. Many people prefer psychological treatments to drug treatments, because they consider (often correctly) that psychological treatments address underlying problems, rather than simply mask superficial symptoms. Of course, drug treatment and psychological treatment are not mutually exclusive and, although psychological treatments can have a role to play in mental disorders such as schizophrenia, bipolar disorder, and severe depression, they are no substitute for treatment with antipsychotic, mood-stabilising, or antidepressant medication. The type of psychological treatment that is chosen, if any, depends not only on your diagnosis but also on your personal circumstances, your preferences, and – sadly all too

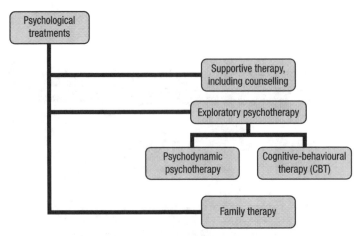

Figure 33.1 The three main forms of psychotherapy: supportive therapy, exploratory psychotherapy, and family therapy. Exploratory psychotherapy can be divided into dynamic therapies based on psychoanalytic theory, and cognitive-behavioural therapies based on learning and cognitive theories. The principal form of the former is psychodynamic psychotherapy, and the principal form of the latter is cognitive-behavioural therapy (CBT).

often – on the funding and human resources that are available in your local area.

At its most basic, psychological treatment involves little more than explanation and reassurance. Such 'supportive therapy' should form an important part of treatment for all mental disorders, and in mild anxiety or depression is often the only treatment that is necessary or, indeed, appropriate. Counselling is similar to supportive therapy in that it involves explanation, reassurance, and support. However, it is more problem-focused and goal-oriented than supportive therapy, as it also involves the identification and resolution of current life difficulties.

In contrast to supportive psychotherapy, exploratory psychotherapy such as cognitive-behavioural therapy (CBT) and psychodynamic psychotherapy aims to delve into the person's thoughts and feelings. Although CBT and psychodynamic psychotherapy are both forms of exploratory psychotherapy, CBT is principally based on learning and cognitive theories, whereas psychodynamic psychotherapy is principally based on psychoanalytic theory. Psychodynamic psychotherapy is similar to psychoanalysis but is briefer and less intensive; it aims to bring unconscious feelings to the surface so that they can be felt and understood, and so 'dealt with'. In contrast to CBT which focuses exclusively on the 'here and now', psychodynamic psychotherapy also focuses on past and childhood experiences, which can particularly useful if the person's problems appear to be rooted there.

Developed by the psychiatrist Aaron Beck (born 1921) in the 1960s, CBT is becoming an increasingly popular form of psychological treatment for a range of mental disorders including anxiety disorders, non-severe depression, eating disorders, and chronic schizophrenia. Compared to psychodynamic psychotherapy, it is more evidence-based and more time-limited, and so more cost-effective. CBT is most often carried out on a one-to-one basis, but can also be offered in small groups. It involves a limited number of sessions, typically between 10 and 20, but principally takes place outside of sessions through 'homework'. The person and a trained therapist (who may be a doctor, a psychologist, a nurse, or a counsellor) develop a shared understanding of the person's current problems and try to understand them in terms of his thoughts (cognitions), emotions, and behaviour, and of how these might be related to one another (Figure 33.2). This then leads to the identification of realistic, time-limited goals, and of cognitive and behavioural strategies for achieving them. For example, in panic disorder these cognitive and behavioural strategies may involve cognitive restructuring (examining, testing, and modifying unhelpful thoughts and beliefs), relaxation training, and graded exposure to anxiety-provoking situations (so-called 'behavioural experiments'). In depression, the principal focus of CBT is to modify automatic and self-perpetuating negative thoughts. These negative thoughts (or 'thinking errors' – see Module 17) are considered to be hypotheses that, through gentle questioning and guided discovery, can be examined, tested, and modified. Behavioural tasks might include self-monitoring, activity scheduling, graded task assignments, and assertiveness training. In some cases, there may also be an added focus on medication compliance and relapse prevention. Many of the self-help techniques in this book are based on cognitive and behavioural strategies used in CBT.

Family therapy involves the identification and resolution of negative aspects of couple or family relationships that may be contributing to mental disorder, such as deeply rooted conflict or high expressed emotion, and usually involves the direct participation of all parties involved. There are also other types of psychological treatment, such as interpersonal therapy (IPT) and dialectical behavioural therapy (DBT). IPT involves a systematic and standardised treatment approach to personal relationships and life problems that are contributing to depression. DBT is a psychological method based on Buddhist teachings for the treatment of borderline personality disorder and recurrent self-harm.

Psychological or 'talking' treatments

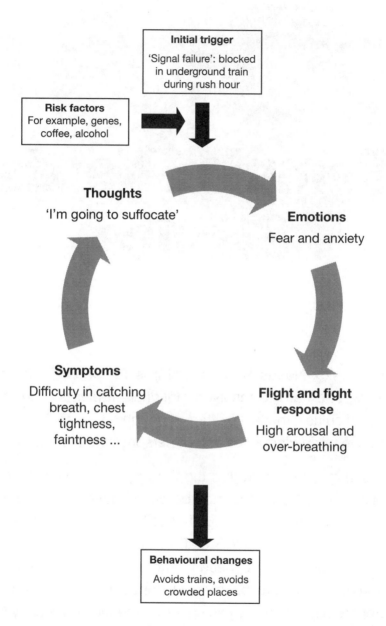

Figure 33.2 This is a CBT model for a person with panic disorder. In CBT, the person and trained therapist develop a shared understanding of the person's current problems and try to understand them in terms of his thoughts, emotions, and behaviour, and of how these might be related to one another.

34
Complex Needs Service

The Complex Needs Service (CNS) is for people with long-standing and hard to resolve emotional problems or interpersonal difficulties; these are often, although not invariably, people who have been diagnosed with a personality disorder.

A person may be referred to the CNS by their psychiatrist, but in many cases he or she may be encouraged to self-refer by calling, writing to, or emailing the CNS. The person then meets with a member of the CNS staff to discuss the CNS and the person's problems and needs. After this initial meeting, the person may decide to join a weekly 'options' group which aims to prepare him or her for joining a therapeutic community (TC). He or she may attend the options group for up to one year, during which time he or she can decide whether or not to join a TC.

Complex Needs Service

Joining a TC involves a commitment to attend a daily programme every weekday for a period of 18 months. This is a
very significant commitment, and demands a very high level of
self-motivation. The idea behind a TC is that a person is best
able to change by interacting positively with other people, that
is, by forming relationships with other people in an atmosphere
of trust and security, and by feeling mutually accepted, valued,
and supported.

A TC is governed by a set of values and beliefs about the way
people should treat each other; these are based on self-aware-
ness, interdependence, deep mutual respect, and the assump-
tion of personal responsibility. There is a busy daily programme
that involves formal and informal therapeutic activities including
group therapy, individual therapy, creative therapies, social or
cultural events, and educational or work placements. Members
also participate in the running of the TC, and may even become
involved in daily activities such as cooking, cleaning, gardening,
and administration. Members and staff meet together regularly
to receive feedback from one another, discuss the running of
the community, and make decisions about it.

People who have spent time in a TC tend to use less medication and healthcare services than they used to, and also tend to
require fewer hospital admissions.

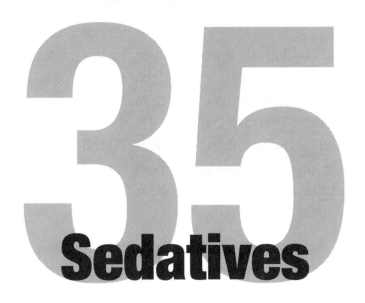
Sedatives

Most sedatives that are prescribed today are benzodiazepines. Benzodiazepines have a range of effects, and they are prescribed not only for difficulty sleeping or insomnia, but also for anxiety, agitation, detoxification from alcohol, convulsions, involuntary movement disorders, spastic disorders, and prior to having a surgical operation.

One of the principal advantages of benzodiazepines is that they start having an effect very quickly. The choice of benzodiazepine is principally determined by its intended use, as potency and duration of action vary considerably from one benzodiazepine to another. For example, temazepam and oxazepam are often chosen for insomnia because, relatively speaking, they have a low potency and a short duration of action, which means that they do not leave people with too many 'hang-over' effects the next day. Other benzodiazepines that you might come across

Sedatives

include alprazolam, clonazepam, diazepam, lorazepam, and chlordiazepoxide.

Common side-effects of benzodiazepines include dizziness, drowsiness, slowing down of movements, difficulty with memory, and – paradoxically – anxiety. If you are taking a benzodiazepine or are still under its effects, you should not drive or operate heavy machinery. Tolerance (meaning that you need progressively higher doses to achieve the same effect) and dependence are major problems with benzodiazepines. As a result, doctors are reluctant to prescribe them, and usually only ever prescribe them in very short courses. Once tolerance has developed, abrupt discontinuation is likely to lead to symptoms such as anxiety and insomnia and, more rarely, to depression, psychosis, seizures, and delirium tremens (see Module 8). While benzodiazepines are relatively safe in overdose, their toxic effects are enhanced by a number of drugs and substances, including alcohol which should definitely be avoided.

36

Antidepressants

What are the different types of antidepressant?

The first antidepressant drug, iproniazid, appeared in the 1950s. Iproniazid was originally trialled in people with tuberculosis, who were subsequently observed to be 'inappropriately happy'. Iproniazid and subsequent drugs in the class of the monoamine oxidase inhibitors (MAOIs) exert their antidepressant effect by preventing the breakdown of monoamine neurotransmitters or 'chemical messengers' in the brain. Back in the 1950s, MAOIs revolutionised the treatment of depression, but people taking them had to comply with a severely restricted diet so as to avoid potentially fatal food reactions. For this and other reasons, MAOIs are seldom used today.

Imipramine, the first tricyclic antidepressant, appeared soon after iproniazid. Although people no longer had to adhere to a severely restricted diet, they continued to suffer from troublesome and potentially dangerous side-effects. Tricyclic antidepressants are effective in the treatment of depression because they prevent the re-uptake of the monoamines neurotransmitters noradrenaline and serotonin by brain cells. While they are still regularly prescribed, their potential side-effects and high toxicity in overdose means that they should be avoided in people who are elderly, physically ill, or at a high risk of committing suicide.

After the late 1950s it took another 30 years for the next class of antidepressants to appear. Fluoxetine, the first serotonin selective reuptake inhibitor (SSRI), only first gained regulatory approval in 1987. Today SSRIs such as fluoxetine, fluvoxamine, paroxetine, sertraline, and citalopram are the treatment of choice for most cases of moderate and severe depression. They are also commonly used in the treatment of a broad range of other mental disorders, particularly anxiety disorders, obsessive-compulsive disorder, and bulimia nervosa. In the UK, fluoxetine is so commonly prescribed that trace quantities have been found in the drinking water. Fluoxetine and other SSRIs prevent the reuptake of the monoamine neurotransmitter serotonin by brain cells. Compared to the older tricyclic antidepressants, SSRIs have milder side-effects and are less toxic in overdose; they are thus particularly useful in people who are elderly, physically ill, or at high risk of committing suicide. Since the 1980s further classes of antidepressants have been developed, such as the noradrenaline reuptake inhibitors (NARIs) and the serotonin and noradrenaline reuptake inhibitors (SNRIs). These more recent classes of antidepressants are often used as second-line treatments if treatment with an SSRI has failed. Commonly prescribed antidepressants are listed in Table 36.1.

Table 36.1: Commonly prescribed antidepressants		
Antidepressant	Trade Name	Licensed daily dose range in adults under the age of 65
Citalopram	Cipramil	20–60mg, tablets or oral drops
Escitalopram	Cipralex	10–20mg, tablets
Fluoxetine	Prozac	20–60mg, tablets or liquid
Fluvoxamine	Faverin	50–300mg, tablets
Paroxetine	Seroxat	20–50mg, tablets or liquid
Sertraline	Lustral	50–200mg, tablets

How should I take my SSRI?

SSRIs are normally taken once a day, in the morning. If you have been prescribed an SSRI, you should be aware that it can take 10–20 days to start having an effect. Your SSRI may initially cause some mild but troublesome side-effects (see later), but these tend to resolve within the first month of treatment. Thus, it is important to stick with your SSRI, even though it may initially seem like it is doing more harm than good. If you fail to respond to your SSRI despite taking it for an adequate length of time, you and your doctor still have several options to choose from, for example, increase the dose, try another SSRI, or try an antidepressant from a different class.

What are the side-effects of SSRIs?

SSRIs, like all medication, can have side-effects, but they are generally less dangerous and better tolerated than those of older types of antidepressants. Common side-effects of SSRIs include nausea, diarrhoea, dizziness, agitation, and sexual dysfunction. With the exception of sexual dysfunction, these tend to resolve within the first month of treatment. Some SSRIs such as fluoxetine, fluvoxamine, and paroxetine inhibit certain enzymes in the liver, and so interfere with the metabolism or breakdown of certain drugs. If you are taking any other drugs, be sure to mention these to your doctor. If an SSRI is suddenly stopped, a discontinuation syndrome consisting of mild and non-specific symptoms can be triggered. This has led to the suggestion that SSRIs are 'addictive', but this is not strictly true in the sense that people do not experience a 'high' from them, and do not seek or crave them as they might a drug of abuse such as cocaine or heroin. It has also been suggested that SSRIs increase suicidal thoughts and behaviour in children and adolescents, but the studies looking into this are equivocal and the jury is still out.

How effective are SSRIs?

Doctors often tell people starting on an SSRI that they have a 55–70 per cent chance of responding to their medication. However, a recent scientific paper in the *New England Journal of Medicine* suggested that the effectiveness of SSRIs has been exaggerated as a result of a bias in the publication of past research studies.

What is the role of antidepressant medication in bipolar disorder?

In bipolar disorder, the most commonly used treatment for a depressive episode is an antidepressant, often in conjunction with a mood stabiliser or an antipsychotic to avoid 'manic switch', that is, over-treatment into mania. If the symptoms of depression are only mild to moderate, it may be preferable to avoid using an antidepressant so as to avoid the risk of manic switch. Once the depressive symptoms have resolved, the antidepressant is tapered off and stopped. In other words, the antidepressant is not continued for the long-term. Other medications that are sometimes used in the treatment of bipolar depression include lithium, valproate, lamotrigine, carbamazepine, or antipsychotic medication (see Modules 37 and 38).

37
Mood stabilisers

Lithium

The Australian psychiatrist and researcher John Cade seren-dipitously discovered the calming properties of lithium in 1948, and the naturally occurring salt became the first effective treat-ment for bipolar disorder. Today lithium is commonly used in the long-term treatment of bipolar disorder to prevent further relapses of both mania and depression, and sometimes also in the short-term treatment of manic and hypomanic episodes. In the long-term treatment of bipolar disorder, it decreases the relapse rates by about one-third, but it is more effective against mania than against depression. Despite its popularity, its mode of action is still unclear. It is understood to have a range of effects on the brain, including effects on certain neurotransmit-ters (or chemical messengers) and their receptors.

Ideally, lithium should be started only if there is a clear intention to continue it for at least three years, since poor compliance and intermittent treatment may precipitate episodes of so-called 'rebound' mania or hypomania. The starting dose of lithium is normally cautious, but depends on the type of preparation used – for example, lithium carbonate versus lithium citrate. A blood test to determine the serum level of lithium needs to be taken about 12 hours after the first dose. Further such blood tests then need to be taken at five to seven day intervals until the serum level of lithium is stable, and thereafter at three- or four-monthly intervals. These blood tests need to be taken because serum lithium levels need to be within a relatively narrow range, or 'therapeutic window', of about 0.5–1.0 millimoles per litre (or 0.8–1.0 millimoles per litre in the short-term treatment of manic and hypomanic episodes). If the serum level of lithium is less than about 0.5 millimoles per litre, beneficial effects are limited; if it is more than about 1.0 millimoles per litre, side-effects and toxic effects are more likely.

The toxic effects of lithium are typically experienced if serum levels exceed 1.5 millimoles per litre. They include anorexia, nausea, vomiting, diarrhoea, coarse tremor, difficulty articulating speech, clumsiness, unsteadiness and, in severe cases, fits and loss of consciousness. Lithium is cleared out of the body through the kidneys, so serum levels of lithium are related to kidney function. For this reason, it is important to check kidney function before lithium is started. This is usually achieved by carrying out a simple blood test.

The side-effects of lithium can occur even when serum lithium levels are within the therapeutic window, and can be divided into short-term and long-term side-effects (see Table 37.1). These are *not* the same as the toxic effects of lithium (see above). Short-term side-effects include a stuffy nose and a metallic taste in the mouth, fine tremor, nausea, diarrhoea, muscle weakness, thirst, and passing a lot of urine. In the long-term, lithium can cause swelling and weight gain, and make certain skin conditions such as acne and psoriasis flare up. Because lithium can affect the thyroid gland and the kidneys, simple blood tests need to be taken at six-monthly intervals to monitor thyroid and kidney function. Lithium can also affect the conduction of electrical impulses in the heart, and for this reason it is standard practice to record a tracing of the heart (an ECG) before starting treatment. If you are pregnant and on lithium, there is a very small chance that lithium might cause a malformation of the heart in the foetus. That having been said, the risk

Table 37.1: Side-effects of lithium	
Short-term	Long-term
Stuffy nose Metallic taste in the mouth Fine tremor Nausea Diarrhoea Muscle weakness Passing a lot of urine ('polyuria') Drinking a lot of water ('polydipsia')	Swelling ('oedema') Weight gain Skin: exacerbation of acne and psoriasis Thyroid: goitre and hypothyroidism Kidneys: renal damage, diabetes insipidus Heart: cardiotoxicity
NB: Before starting on lithium it is standard practice to take a simple blood test to check kidney and thyroid function, and to record a tracing of the heart.	

of this happening is less than one in 1,000, and this risk needs to be counterbalanced against the much higher risk of relapse if lithium is stopped or if the dose is decreased. As lithium is passed into breast milk, breast-feeding should be avoided.

Lithium has a response rate of about 75 per cent in the treatment of short-term manic and hypomanic episodes, but it takes several days to produce an effect. If lithium is effective and side-effects are absent or tolerable, it should be continued in the long-term. If not, it can be stopped abruptly. In contrast, after long-term treatment it should only be stopped gradually, over the course of two to three months, to minimise the risk of precipitating an episode of rebound mania or hypomania. People who are on lithium should drink plenty of fluids and avoid reducing their salt intake, because dehydration and salt depletion can in some cases precipitate lithium toxicity.

Valproate, lamotrigine, and carbamazepine

The use of anticonvulsants (principally valproate and, more recently, lamotrigine) in the long-term treatment of bipolar disorder is increasing. However, their precise mode of action in preventing relapses of bipolar disorder is as yet unclear.

Valproate, in the form of semisodium valproate (Depakote), is used alone or as an adjunct to lithium or other medications in the long-term and short-term treatment of bipolar disorder, and in the USA it has become the most frequently prescribed mood stabiliser. Compared with lithium, it has similar efficacy but a quicker onset of action. It is also of particular value in rapid-cycling bipolar disorder, a particularly severe form of bipolar disorder that involves four or more episodes of mania, hypomania, depression, or mixed states in a period of one year. Although valproate can have a number of side-effects, it is often better tolerated than lithium, particularly if lithium levels need to be maintained above 0.8 millimoles per litre. Side-effects of valproate include nausea, tremor, tiredness, weight gain, hair loss, blood cell problems, and liver toxicity. During pregnancy, valproate can significantly increase the risk of malformations in the foetus; for this reason, it may be avoided in women of child-bearing age. It is important to check blood cell counts and liver function before valproate is started, and to continue monitoring these at six- to twelve-monthly intervals. This is usually achieved by carrying out a simple blood test.

In contrast to lithium, lamotrigine is more effective against relapses of depression than against relapses of mania, and it can be used both as a short-term treatment for relapses of depression and for long-term mood stabilisation. Compared with the other mood stabilisers discussed in this module, lamotrigine has fewer side-effects and does not usually require long-term monitoring with blood tests. However, monitoring of serum levels of lamotrigine may be required if it is being taken in combination with either valproate or carbamazepine because both of these affect the metabolism (or breakdown) of lamotrigine. Common side-effects include nausea and vomiting, dizziness, clumsiness and unsteadiness, sedation, and insomnia. Other side-effects include irritation of the oesophagus (or food pipe), blurred vision, skin rash, and severe skin reactions.

Carbamazepine may be used as a second- or third-line treatment in the long-term treatment of bipolar disorder, and is thought to be of particular value in treatment-resistant cases and in rapid-cycling. Side-effects include nausea, headache, dizziness, tiredness, double vision, clumsiness and unsteadiness, skin rashes, electrolyte disturbances, blood cell problems, and liver toxicity. Blood tests need to be taken regularly to monitor liver function, blood cell counts, and electrolytes. If used in pregnancy, carbamazepine can result in malformations of the foetus, but it is not excreted in breast milk and can be used even if breast-feeding. Carbamazepine activates certain enzymes in the liver and so speeds up the metabolism (or breakdown) of a number of other drugs such as antipsychotics, lamotrigine, and the oral contraceptive pill. If you are about to start on carbamazepine, you should tell your doctor about any other drugs that you are taking.

Which mood stabiliser should I choose?

Your choice of mood stabiliser should ideally depend on several factors, including:

- The type of symptoms that you have.

- Your response to previous treatments, if any.

- Your physical health, for instance, the presence of obesity, diabetes, or kidney disease.

- Your degree of motivation and level of compliance with medication.

- Your personal preference.

- Your psychiatrist's opinion.

What if my chosen mood stabiliser does not work for me?

If you have frequent relapses despite being on a mood stabiliser, you can either change to a different mood stabiliser or start taking a second mood stabiliser in addition to the first one (for example, start taking valproate in addition to lithium). Should you start on such combination therapy, symptoms, side-effects, and serum levels should be very closely monitored. If you continue having frequent relapses on combination therapy, your psychiatrist may refer you to a clinician with particular expertise in the treatment of bipolar disorder for a so-called 'second opinion'.

38
Antipsychotics

How effective are antipsychotics in the treatment of schizophrenia?

Antipsychotics are effective in the treatment of the positive symptoms of schizophrenia principally because they block the effects of increased dopamine in a part of the brain called the mesolimbic tract. Antipsychotics are effective in controlling positive symptoms in about 70–80 per cent of people with schizophrenia, although it often takes several days before any effects are evident. Until then a person with schizophrenia may benefit from taking a sedative such as lorazepam if he or she is distressed or agitated. In some cases, several antipsychotics may need to be tried before the one that is best for him or her can be found, and this involves an inevitable period of 'trial and error'. Unfortunately, antipsychotic medication has relatively little effect on the cognitive and negative symptoms of schizophrenia. Note that antipsychotics are also commonly used for the treatment of other mental disorders, particularly bipolar disorder and other psychotic disorders.

Are antipsychotics always needed in the treatment of schizophrenia?

Although non-pharmacological, psychosocial treatments have an important role to play in the management of schizophrenia, antipsychotic medication is always needed. Indeed, scientific research has conclusively demonstrated that long-term antipsychotic treatment reduces rates of relapse and re-hospitalisation in a substantial number of people with schizophrenia. Many people understandably do not like taking too much medication, because they are frightened of becoming addicted to pills, or frightened of suffering from undesirable side-effects. Like all medication, antipsychotic medication can have side-effects, but it is not in any sense addictive. Adequate management of the situation involves balancing the risks and benefits of treatment with antipsychotic medication, and reassessing that balance in light of changing circumstances. It is important to remember that not all people taking antipsychotic medication suffer from side-effects, and that, for many of those who do, the side-effects are only mild or temporary.

Which antipsychotic should I choose?

Current treatment guidelines for the treatment of schizophrenia recommend starting on one of the more recent ('atypical') antipsychotics, which, compared with the older ('typical') antipsychotics, are less likely to produce disturbances of voluntary muscle function called extrapyramidal side-effects (see later). There are several atypical antipsychotics, and risperidone, olanzapine, and quetiapine are among the most commonly prescribed ones. While these antipsychotics are on balance similarly effective, each has a slightly different side-effect profile. In addition, some antipsychotics come in different forms that can make taking them easier. For example, they may come in liquid form or as an oral dispersible tablet (ODT) that dissolves in the mouth. While sharing experiences can be useful, it is important not to be overly influenced by other people's individual experiences with one or another antipsychotic. Every person is unique, and for this reason there is no one antipsychotic that best suits all. The various factors involved in choosing an antipsychotic are listed in Table 38.1.

Table 38.1: Principal factors involved in choosing an antipsychotic
Initially Particular side-effects that you are keen to avoid Previous side-effects that you have found to be unacceptable Difficulties that you anticipate in taking the tablet in its standard tablet form
Later in the course of treatment Effectiveness of the antipsychotic at controlling your symptoms Current side-effects that you find unacceptable Difficulties that you are having in taking the tablet in its standard tablet form

What are the side-effects of antipsychotic medication?

Antipsychotics are effective in the treatment of the positive symptoms of schizophrenia because they block the effects of increased dopamine in the mesolimbic tract. Unfortunately, they can also block the effects of dopamine in other brain tracts, leading to a number of potential side-effects such as negative symptoms, disturbances of voluntary muscle function called extrapyramidal side-effects, loss of libido, and erectile dysfunction. Antipsychotic drugs can also interfere with other neurotransmitters in the brain, and this may potentially result in further side-effects such as sedation and weight gain, which are both common. Weight gain can place you at long-term risk of heart disease and diabetes, so if you are on antipsychotic medication it is particularly important that you have your physical health monitored, avoid smoking, develop and maintain healthy eating habits, and take regular exercise. Other common side-effects of antipsychotic medication include orthostatic hypotension (dizziness upon sitting up and standing), and so-called 'anticholinergic side-effects' such as dry mouth, blurred vision, and constipation. There are four different types of extrapyramidal side-effect, as detailed in Table 38.2. Any side-effects that have not been mentioned are comparatively uncommon or may vary from one antipsychotic to another.

What is Aripiprazole?

Aripiprazle is a novel, so-called 'third-generation' antipsychotic that has been described as a 'dopamine-serotonin system sta-

Table 38.2: Extrapyramidal side-effects of antipsychotic medication	
Acute dystonia	Painful contraction of a muscle or muscle group, most commonly in the neck, eyes, and trunk. They are easy to recognise and manage
Akathisia	Distressing feeling of inner restlessness manifested by fidgety leg movements, shuffling of the feet, and pacing. Management usually involves reducing the dose of the antipsychotic or changing to another antipsychotic
Parkinson-like symptoms	Tremor, muscular rigidity, and difficulty starting movements. Management usually involves reducing the dose of the antipsychotic or changing to another antipsychotic
Tardive dyskinesia	Involuntary, repetitive, and purposeless movements of the tongue, lips, face, trunk, and extremities, usually occurring after several years of antipsychotic treatment. The movements may be generalised or only affect certain muscle groups, typically the muscles around the mouth. Management is very difficult

biliser'. It is purported to have good efficacy in treating positive symptoms, negative symptoms, and mood symptoms, and to be better tolerated than other antipsychotics. Principal side-effects include headache, anxiety, insomnia, nausea, vomiting, and light-headedness but *not* extrapyramidal side-effects, sexual side-effects, sedation, or weight gain.

Antipsychotics in pregnancy and breast-feeding

There is some scientific data to suggest that exposure to an antipsychotic during the first trimester of pregnancy is linked to a small additional risk of congenital abnormalities in the foetus. However, withholding the antipsychotic may result in behavioural disturbances that expose the mother and foetus to much higher levels of overall risk. For this reason, pregnant women are generally advised to remain on their antipsychotic for the full duration of their pregnancy.

Antipsychotics are excreted into breast milk but, except in the case of clozapine, breast-fed infants do not seem to suffer from this. For this reason, a mother may decide to breast-feed while remaining on her antipsychotic.

Starting antipsychotic medication

The starting dose of an antipsychotic is usually small so as to minimise any potential side-effects. The dose is then increased according to the person's response, up to the minimum dose that is effective for that person. This dose varies according to a large number of factors, including age, sex, and weight.

If a person does not respond to the chosen antipsychotic after a trial period of six to eight weeks, the antipsychotic can be stopped and a different one started. If a person does not respond to two or more antipsychotics, the atypical antipsychotic clozapine can be considered. Although clozapine is particularly effective in treatment-resistant schizophrenia, it requires registration with a monitoring service and, in the initial period, daily monitoring of vital signs as well as weekly blood tests. The blood tests monitor the white cell count, which can drop dangerously in up to 1 per cent of people on clozapine. The role of white blood cells is to fight infections, so a drop in the white cell count can suddenly leave the body exposed to danger.

For how long should an antipsychotic be taken?

Antipsychotics not only control the symptoms of schizophrenia, but also make them less likely to re-occur. If you have improved on a particular antipsychotic, you should continue taking it at the same dose for *at least* the next six months, preferably for the next 12 to 24 months, and possibly for considerably longer.

What is a depot antipsychotic?

Some people who have difficulties taking their antipsychotic may benefit from receiving it in the form of an injectable long-term preparation, or 'depot', instead of the usual oral tablet or oral liquid form. The principal advantages and disadvantages of depot versus oral antipsychotic medication are listed in Table 38.3. Before starting a person on a depot, it is usual to first administer an oral test dose. After about seven days, the first depot dose is administered, and the dose is then increased at regular intervals as the oral antipsychotic is decreased and stopped. Depot injections are usually given every 7 or 14 days. The commonly used typical, atypical, and depot antipsychotics are listed in Table 38.4.

Table 38.3: Principal advantages and disadvantages of oral versus depot antipsychotics

	Advantages	Disadvantages
Oral medication	Short duration of action Flexible	Variable absorption from the gut Potential for poor compliance Potential for misuse/ overdose
Depot medication	Less potential for poor compliance Less potential for misuse/overdose Regular contact with health worker	Needle injections Potential delayed side-effects Potential prolonged side-effects

Table 38.4: Commonly used atypical, typical, and depot antipsychotics

Antipsychotic medication	Trade name	Licensed daily dose range in adults under the age of 65
Atypical antipsychotics (introduced from 1990)		
Olanzapine	Zyprexa	15–20mg
Quetiapine	Seroquel	100–800mg (usual dose range 400–800mg)
Clozapine*	Clozaril, Denzapine	25–900mg (usual dose range 200–450mg)
Risperidone	Risperdal	2–16mg (rarely exceeds 10mg)
Amisulpiride	Solian	400–1200mg
Aripiprazole	Abilify	10–30mg
		continued overleaf

Table 38.4: Commonly used atypical, typical, and depot antipsychotics – *contd*		
Antipsychotic medication	Trade name	Licensed daily dose range in adults under the age of 65
Typical antipsychotics (introduced from the 1950s)		
Chlorpromazine	Largactil	75–1000mg
Fluphenazine	Modecate/Moditen	2–20mg
Haloperidol	Haldol/Dozic/ Serenace	3–30mg
Pimozide	Orap	2–20mg
Flupenthixol	Depixol	3–18mg
Zuclopenthixol	Clopixol	20–150mg
Sulpiride	Dolmatil/Sulpitil/ Sulpor	400–2400mg
Depot antipsychotics		
Risperidone	Risperdal Consta	Maximum dose: 50mg every 2 weeks
Fluphenazine decanoate	Modecate	Test dose: 12.5mg; maximum dose: 100mg every 2 weeks
Flupenthixol decanoate	Depixol	Test dose: 20mg; maximum dose: 400mg per week
Zuclopenthixol decanoate	Clopixol	Test dose: 100mg; maximum dose: 600mg per week
Pipiotazine palmitate	Piportil depot	Test dose: 25mg; maximum: 200mg every 4 weeks

39 Taking your medication

Some people with a mental disorder, particularly a psychotic illness, may be reluctant to take their prescribed medication because they do not realise or accept that they are ill. Other common reasons for not taking medication include fear of side-effects, fear of addiction, poor concentration or motivation, delusional beliefs about the medication (for example, that it is poison), or a poor relationship with the prescribing doctor or with another member of the mental healthcare team. Some people may also stop taking their medication because they have made a good recovery and feel that the medication is no longer needed.

Stopping your prescribed medication or even occasionally missing tablets can lead to a relapse or recurrence of symptoms. If you suffer from a psychotic illness, taking your medication in the manner prescribed is often the single most important thing that you can do to prevent a relapse. After each relapse, it may become increasingly difficult for you to regain control over your symptoms. For this reason, it is particularly important for both you and your family to discuss any difficulties in taking your medication and to have these difficulties addressed in as far as is possible. For example, your doctor may be able to simplify your medication schedule, reduce the dose of your medication, change you medication to a different one, or simply provide you with advice or reassurance. *Do not simply stop taking your medication*.

You may find it helpful to keep a treatment diary in which you record the names of the different medications that you have taken, their benefits, and any side-effects. Such a treatment diary can help you and your doctor to choose the most suitable medication for you. Figure 39.1 is an example of such a treatment diary.

For specific information on drugs commonly prescribed in the treatment of mental disorders, see Modules 35–38.

Medication	Dates taken	How taken	Benefits	Side-effects
Risperidone	15/01/08–30/03/08	Tablets Once a day	* Voices almost disappeared * Felt more relaxed * Easy to take	* Felt tired all day long * Felt dizzy on standing
Olanzapine	30/03/08 to present	Tablets Once a day	* Voices fully controlled * Feel even more relaxed than on risperidone * Easy to take	Initially put on 3kg (I have since lost this weight through diet and exercise)

Figure 39.1 My treatment diary

Electroconvulsive therapy

Although electroconvulsive therapy (ECT) still has a poor public image, it has been scientifically demonstrated to be safe and effective in the treatment of mood symptoms that are both severe and unresponsive to medication. It is typically prescribed for people with severe depression who are at an ongoing high risk to themselves, either because of profound suicidal ideation, psychotic symptoms such as hallucinations and delusions, retardation or stupor, or food refusal.

How does ECT work?

According to the original monoamine hypothesis of depression, depression results from the depletion of the monoamine neurotransmitters serotonin, noradrenaline, and dopamine in the brain. In its revised, modern version the monoamine hypothesis recognises that depression may not result from an actual depletion of monoamine neurotransmitters, but from a change in their receptors' function. The principal source of support for the monoamine hypothesis comes from the various antidepressant drugs, which act in different ways to increase the levels of one or more monoamine neurotransmitters in the brain. ECT has been found to alter the receptors for the monoamine neurotransmitter serotonin, but its precise mechanism of action in the treatment of depression is still unclear.

Are there any contraindications to ECT?

ECT is a potentially life-saving treatment, and its risks and benefits need to be weighed up for each individual person. While there are no absolute contraindications to ECT, relative contraindications include cardiovascular disease, dementia, epilepsy and other neurological disorders, raised intracranial pressure (for example, as a result of a head injury or brain tumour), and cervical spine disease. Pregnancy and old age are not contraindications to ECT.

Is any preparation required before starting ECT?

Prior to starting a course of ECT, a person should have a physical examination, a tracting of the heart (ECG), and some blood tests, and should not eat or drink (unless as instructed, for instance, to take medication) from the previous midnight. Informed consent is needed except if being treated under the provision of the Mental Health Act. The Mental Act 2007 (see Module 44) introduces new safeguards for the use of ECT. In short, ECT may not be given to a person with the capacity to refuse to consent to it, and it may only be given to a person without the capacity to refuse consent to it if this does not conflict with any advance directive, decision of a donee or deputy, or decision of the Court of Protection.

How is ECT delivered?

During ECT treatment the person is given a standard anaesthetic and a muscle relaxant. The seizure is induced by delivering a constant current, brief-pulse stimulus at a voltage that is just above the person's seizure threshold. The seizure typically lasts for about 30 seconds, and in many cases it is so small that it can barely be seen other than on an electroencephalograph (EEG) monitor. Most people respond to a course of between six and twelve ECT treatments, which are usually delivered over the course of three to six weeks.

What are the side effects of ECT?

Side-effects of ECT include nausea, muscle aches, headache, confusion, and memory loss for events that occurred around the time of treatment and, less frequently, in the more distant past. Memories for events that occurred in the more distant past may later be recovered, and many people undergoing ECT treatment actually feel their memory improving as the treatment takes effect, the depression lifts, and the ability to concentrate returns. Mortality from ECT is largely imputable to the anaesthetic, and is thus similar to that for any minor surgical procedure.

Section 5

Mental health services and the law

41 A guide to mental healthcare services

Some 40 or 50 years ago, many if not most people with a first episode of a serious mental illness such as schizophrenia would have been admitted to a psychiatric hospital for assessment and treatment, and some may have remained as in-patients for an indefinitely long period of time. In the 1950s and 1960s this so-called 'institutional model' of psychiatric care came under heavy criticism for isolating and institutionalising people with mental disorders, and thereby condoning their stigmatisation by 'mainstream' society. This led to a trend of removing people with mental disorder from psychiatric hospitals in the hope of integrating them into the community. This trend, greatly facilitated by the advent of the first psychiatric drugs in the 1950s and 1960s, continued throughout the 1970s and 1980s.

The advantages of community care are clear. By shifting the emphasis from a person's mental disorder to his or her strengths and life aspirations, community care promotes independence and self-reliance, while discouraging isolation and institution-alisation and reducing stigmatisation. That having been said, a lack of mental health staff and resources can in some cases shift the burden of care onto informal carers such as relatives and friends, and make it especially difficult to care for those most in need of care, such as the isolated or the homeless.

Organisation of mental healthcare services

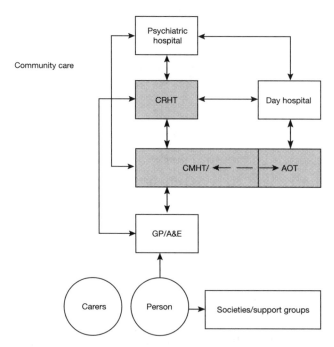

Figure 41.1 Example of organisation of mental healthcare services (your local services may differ). Note that mental healthcare services are organised to facilitate community care and avoid unnecessary hospital admissions. All terms used in this figure are explained in this module. CRHT, Crisis Resolution and Home Treatment Team; CMHT, Community Mental Health Team; EIS, Early Intervention Services; AOT or AORT, Assertive Outreach Team; GP – general practitioner (or family doctor); A&E, Accident and Emergency Department.

General practice and A&E

If a person is suffering from the symptoms of a mental disorder, the first port of call is usually the family doctor or general practitioner (GP). If the GP forms an opinion that a person might be suffering from a severe mental disorder, he or she is most likely to refer the person to specialist services – either to their local Community Mental Health Team (CMHT) or, in an emergency, to the Crisis Resolution and Home Treatment Team (CRHT).

Some people suffering with the symptoms of a mental disorder first present to A&E instead of to their GP. In this case they are usually screened by a casualty doctor, and then referred for assessment by a psychiatrist. Again, if the psychiatrist forms an opinion that a person might be suffering from a severe mental disorder, he or she is most likely to refer the person to their local CMHT or, in an emergency, to the CRHT.

Community Mental Health Team and Assertive Outreach Team

The CMHT is at the centre of mental healthcare provision. It is a multidisciplinary team led by a consultant psychiatrist and operating from a team base close to the patients that it serves. Community psychiatric nurses (CPNs) and social workers are key members of the CMHT, and often take a lead in implementing and co-ordinating a person's care and treatment plan, and in monitoring his or her progress in the community. Other important members of the CMHT include psychiatrists, clinical psychologists, occupational therapists, pharmacists, and administrative staff (see Table 41.1).

If a person is referred to a CMHT, he or she usually undergoes an initial assessment by a psychiatrist, sometimes in the presence of another member of the team, such as a CPN or social worker. The skill mix of the multidisciplinary team means that the different parts of the person's life can be understood – and addressed – from a number of different angles.

Some people are reluctant to seek help and treatment, and as a consequence appear at the CMHT only in times of crisis. Paradoxically, these people often have the most complex mental health needs and social problems. For this reason, the responsibility for their care is sometimes transferred to the Assertive Outreach Team (AOT), a specialised multidisciplinary team dedicated to engaging them in treatment and supporting them in their daily activities.

Table 41.1: Key members of the CMHT	
Psychiatrist	The psychiatrist is a medical doctor who specialises in diagnosing and treating mental disorders such as schizophrenia, bipolar disorder, depression, and anxiety disorders. The psychiatrist takes a lead role in making a diagnosis and formulating a care and treatment plan
Community psychiatric nurse (CPN)	The CPN is the member of the team that a person under the care of a CMHT is likely to come into contact with most often. The CPN usually visits him or her to monitor progress and facilitate the care and treatment plan

Table 41.1: Key members of the CMHT – *contd*	
Social worker	Sometimes a person under the care of a CMHT may be allocated a social worker instead of, or as well as, a CPN. In the former case, the social worker fulfils a role similar to that of the CPN. The social worker can also help to sort out housing and benefits and ensure that the person makes the most of any services and facilities that are available
Clinical psychologist	'Psychologist' is often confused with 'psychiatrist'. Whereas a psychiatrist is a medical doctor specialising in the diagnosis and treatment of mental illnesses, a psychologist has expertise in human experience and behaviour. A psychologist may spend time listening to and trying to understand a person with a mental disorder and his or her carers. A psychologist may also carry out talking treatments such as cognitive behavioural therapy or family therapy
Occupational therapist	The role of the occupational therapist is to help a person with a mental disorder to maintain his or her skills as well as to develop new ones. This not only helps him or her to get back to work, but also keeps him or her engaged and motivated. Unfortunately, owing to limited resources, many people who come under the care of a CMHT are not allocated an occupational therapist
	continued overleaf

Table 41.1: Key members of the CMHT – *contd*	
Pharmacist	People with a mental disorder who also have a physical illness or who are pregnant or breast-feeding may find it particularly useful to speak to a pharmacist who can help with information about medication
Administrative staff	Administrative staff are responsible for arranging appointments and serve as a crucial point of contact for people with a mental disorder and other members of the team
NB: Other forms of support that are available but that do not form part of the CMHT include support groups, telephone helplines, and the Citizens Advice Bureau.	

Early Intervention Service

Like the AOT, the Early Intervention Service (EIS) may also operate from the CMHT base. Its role is specifically to improve the short-term and long-term outcomes of schizophrenia and schizophrenia-like psychotic disorders through a three-pronged approach involving preventative measures, earlier detection of untreated cases, and intensive treatment and support at the beginning of the illness.

Crisis Resolution and Home Treatment Team

The CRHT, or 'crisis team' for short, is a 24-hours-a-day, 365-days-a-year multidisciplinary team that in some services acts as a gatekeeper to a variety of psychiatric services, including admission to a psychiatric hospital. People with acute mental health problems are referred to the CRHT from a variety of places and agencies, most commonly GPs, A&E, and CMHTs. A member of the team (often a CPN) promptly assesses the person in conjunction with a psychiatrist to determine if a hospital admission can be avoided by providing short-term intensive home care. If so, the CRHT arranges for a member of the team to visit the person's home up to three times a day, gradually decreasing the frequency of visits as the person gets better. Other than simply providing support, the CHRT can assist in implementing a care and treatment plan and in monitoring progress. If a person has already been admitted to hospital, the CRHT can also be involved in expediting and facilitating his or her discharge back into the community. The key features of the CRHT are summarised in Table 41.2.

Table 41.2: Key features of the Crisis Resolution and Home Treatment Team

- Gatekeeper to mental health services, including admission to a psychiatric hospital
- Prompt assessment of a person in a crisis
- Intensive, community-based, round-the-clock support in the early stages of the crisis
- Continued involvement until the crisis has resolved
- Work to prevent similar crises from occurring again
- Partnership with the person and his or her relatives and carers

---

Psychiatric hospital and day hospital

If a person with a mental disorder is admitted to hospital this is usually because care in the community is not an option. Possible reasons for admission to a psychiatric hospital are summarised in Table 41.3.

Table 41.3: Possible reasons for admission to a psychiatric hospital

- Safety of the person with a mental disorder, his or her carers, or the general public
- Management of acute exacerbations, for example, severe psychotic symptoms
- Management of physical complications, for example, malnutrition
- Stabilisation of medication
- Establishment of a diagnosis
- Alternative to community care if adequate support is lacking
- Respite for relatives or carers

Of the small minority of people with a mental disorder who need to be admitted to a psychiatric hospital, the majority are admitted on a voluntary basis. This is either because they are happy to take the advice of their psychiatrist or carers, or because they are frightened of their symptoms and feel that the psychiatric hospital is a safe place for them to be in. In some cases, attendance at a day hospital during office hours of approximately 9.00 a.m. to 5.00 p.m. may provide a more tolerable alternative to hospital admission.

A minority of people with a mental disorder who need to be admitted to a psychiatric hospital refuse to be admitted, usually because they lack insight into their mental disorder and do not think that they are mentally ill. In most countries there are special legal provisions to protect such people from the consequences of their mental disorder. In England and Wales, provisions for compulsory admission and treatment of mental disorders are made by the Mental Health Act 1983. The equivalent legislation on Scotland is the Mental Health (Care and Treatment) Act 2003, and in Northern Ireland it is the Mental Health (Northern Ireland) Order 1986.

The care programme approach

The longer-term care and treatment of people accepted into specialist mental healthcare services is usually planned at one or several Care Programme Approach (CPA) meetings usually attended by both the person with a mental disorder and his or her carers. These meetings are useful for establishing the context of the person's illness; evaluating his or her current personal circumstances; assessing his or her medical, psychological, and social needs; and formulating a detailed care and treatment plan to ensure that these needs are met. As well as ensuring that the person takes his or her medication and is regularly seen by a psychiatrist, CPN, or social worker, this care and treatment plan may involve a number of psychological or social interventions such as attendance at self-help groups, carer education and support, home help, and cognitive-behavioural therapy. A care co-ordinator, most often a CPN or social worker, is appointed to ensure that the care and treatment plan is implemented and revised in light of changing needs and circumstances. The sorts of people who regularly attend CPA meetings are listed in Table 42.1.

Table 42.1: The sorts of people who regularly attend CPA meetings

- The person with a mental disorder
- His or her relatives, carers, or advocates
- The Responsible Clinician (usually a consultant psychiatrist)
- Other psychiatrists
- The GP
- The care co-ordinator (most often a CPN or social worker)

At the outcome of a CPA meeting, the person with a mental disorder should feel that his or her circumstances and needs have been understood, and that the care and treatment plan that he or she has helped to formulate closely reflects these.

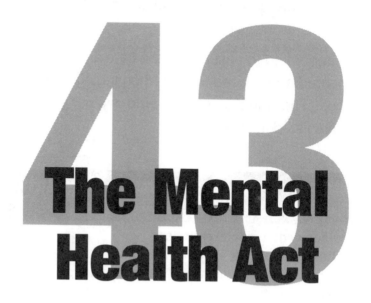

The Mental Health Act

In England and Wales, the Mental Health Act is the principal Act governing not only the compulsory admission and detention of people to a psychiatric hospital, but also their treatment, discharge from hospital, and aftercare. People with a mental disorder as defined by the Act can be detained under the Act in the interests of their health or safety or in the interests of the safety of others. To minimise the potential for abuse, the Act specifically excludes as mental disorder promiscuity, other 'immoral' conduct, sexual deviancy, and dependence on alcohol or drugs. Note that Scotland is governed by the Mental Health (Care and Treatment) (Scotland) Act 2003 and Northern Ireland by the Mental Health (Northern Ireland) Order 1986.

What is a 'section 2'?

Two of the most common 'sections' of the Mental Health Act that are used to admit people with a mental disorder to a psychiatric hospital are the so-called sections 2 and 3. Section 2 allows for an admission for assessment and treatment that can last for up to 28 days. An application for a section 2 is usually made by an Approved Mental Health Professional (AMHP) with special training in mental health, and recommended by two doctors, one of whom must have special experience in the diagnosis and treatment of mental disorders. Under a section 2, treatment can be given, but only if this treatment is aimed at treating the mental disorder or conditions directly resulting from the mental disorder (so, for example, treatment for an inflamed appendix cannot be given under the Act, although treatment for deliberate self-harm might). A section 2 can be 'discharged' or revoked at any time by the Responsible Clinician (usually the consultant psychiatrist in charge), by the hospital managers, or by the nearest relative. Furthermore, a person under a section 2 can appeal against the section, in which case his or her appeal is heard by a specially constituted tribunal. The claimant is represented by a solicitor who helps him or her to make a case in favour of discharge to the tribunal. The tribunal is by nature adversarial, and it falls upon members of the detained person's care team to argue the case for continued detention. This can be quite trying for both the claimant and his or her care team, and it can at times undermine the claimant's trust in the care team.

What is a 'section 3'?

A person can be detained under a 'section 3' after a conclusive period of assessment under a section 2. Alternatively, he or she can be detained directly under a section 3 if his or her diagnosis has already been established by the care team and is not in reasonable doubt. Section 3 corresponds to an admission for treatment and lasts for up to six months. As for a section 2, it is usually applied for by an AMHP with special training in mental health and approved by two doctors, one of whom must have special experience in the diagnosis and treatment of mental disorders. Treatment can only be given under a section 3 if it is aimed at treating the mental disorder or conditions directly resulting from the mental disorder. After the first three months, any treatment requires either the consent of the person being treated or the recommendation of a second doctor. A section 3 can be discharged at any time by the Responsible Clinician (usually the consultant psychiatrist in charge), by the hospital managers, or by the nearest relative. Furthermore, the person under a section 3 can appeal against the section, in which case his or her appeal is heard by a specially constituted tribunal, as explained above. If the person still needs to be detained after six months, the section 3 can be renewed for a further period.

What is 'aftercare'?

If a person has been detained under section 3 of the Mental Health Act, he or she is automatically placed under a 'section 117' at the time of his or her discharge from the section 3. Section 117 corresponds to 'aftercare' and places a duty on the local health authority and local social services authority to provide the person with a care package aimed at rehabilitation and relapse prevention. Although the person is under no obligation to accept aftercare, in some cases he or she may also be placed under 'Supervised Community Treatment' or

Guardianship to ensure that he or she receives aftercare. Under Supervised Community Treatment, the person is made subject to certain conditions; if these conditions are not met, he or she can be recalled into hospital.

44 Driving and DVLA regulations

The following advice applies to mania, schizophrenia and other schizophrenia-like psychotic disorders, and more severe forms of anxiety and depression.

You should stop driving during a first episode or relapse of your illness, because driving while ill can seriously endanger lives. In the UK, you must notify the Driver and Vehicle Licensing Authority (DVLA). Failure to do so makes it illegal for you to drive and invalidates your insurance. The DVLA then sends you a medical questionnaire to fill in, and a form asking for your permission to contact your psychiatrist. Your driving license can generally be reinstated if your psychiatrist can confirm that:

- Your illness has been successfully treated with medication for a variable period of time, typically at least three months.

- You are conscientious about taking your medication.

- The side-effects of your medication are not likely to impair your driving.

- You are not misusing drugs.

People who suffer from substance misuse or dependence should also stop driving, as should some people who suffer from other mental disorders such as dementia, learning disability, or personality disorder. If you are in any doubt as to whether this advice applies to you, speak to your GP or psychiatrist at the soonest opportunity.

Further information can be obtained from the DVLA website at www.DVLA.gov.uk. Note that the rules for professional driving are different from those described above.

45

Social benefits

Every year in the UK millions of pounds of benefits are left unclaimed, often by people with a mental disorder and their carers. Some of the benefits available to people with a mental disorder and their carers are detailed here. For further information on these benefits, see the Department for Work and Pensions website, www.dwp.gov.uk/lifeevent/benefit, contact your local Citizens Advice Bureau, or get in touch with local Social Services.

Housing benefit and council tax benefit

Housing benefit and council tax benefit are means-tested, tax-free payments made to people who need help paying their rent and their council tax, respectively. Both benefits are administered by the local authority in whose area the property is situated. These benefits do not cover mortgage interest payments.

Income support

Income support is a means-tested payment made to people who are between the ages of 16 and 59, who work fewer than 16 hours a week, and who have a reason for not actively seeking work (on the grounds of disability, caring for children, or caring for relatives). Claimants of income support are also entitled to other benefits such as housing benefit and council tax benefit (see above).

Social fund

Social fund payments are payments, grants, or loans made in addition to certain benefits for important intermittent expenses that cannot be met by normal income.

Incapacity benefit

Incapacity benefit is paid to people who cannot work because of illness or disability and who cannot get statutory sick pay from their employer. It is related to national insurance contributions and requires regular medical certificates. It is not means-tested.

Disabled person's tax credit

The disabled person's tax credit is for people over the age of 16 who work an average of 16 hours a week or more, and who have an illness or disability that restricts the amount that they can earn.

Disability living allowance

Disability living allowance is paid to people under the age of 65 who are in need of personal care or help with getting around, or both. It is not means-tested.

Attendance allowance

Attendance allowance is paid to people aged 65 or more who need help with personal care because of an illness or disability. It is not means-tested.

NHS costs

Depending on your circumstances you may qualify for free NHS prescriptions and hospital medicines, free NHS dental treatment, and free NHS eyesight tests. Other NHS costs may be met too.

Carer's allowance

Carer's allowance is a means-tested, taxable weekly bene-fit payment made to people who look after someone who is

Social benefits

receiving Attendance Allowance or Disability Living Allowance at the middle or high rate of care. Among other stipulations, the carer must be over 16 years of age and spend 35 hours a week or more in his or her caring role. The carer does not have to be related to or living with the person whom he or she is caring for.

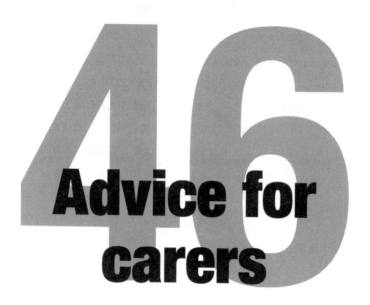

Advice for carers

According to Carers UK, each year in the UK over two million people take up a caring role, so as a carer you are certainly not alone. An attentive carer can be the most valuable source of structure and support for a person with a mental disorder, and his or her greatest hope for a permanent recovery. Although you may feel that caring for a loved one is more a duty than a job, it is important that you identify yourself as a carer so as to obtain the help and support that all people in a caring role are entitled to.

Try to learn as much as you can about the mental disorder of your loved one, so that you have a good idea of how it might be affecting him or her. For example, he or she may lack spontaneity when replying to your questions. This may be because he or she is being distracted by voices or otherwise unable to concentrate, rather than because he or she is ignoring you.

Advice for carers

Understanding the illness builds up your confidence as a carer and gives you a clearer sense of what you may or may not be able to achieve. Remember that there is only so much you alone can do to help your loved one: being realistic about how much you can achieve enables you to prevent conflict, manage stress, and avoid burn-out. Speak to your local mental health-care team for further information about the mental disorder of your loved one, and for specific advice on caring for him or her. Information and advice is also available from voluntary organi-sations such as those listed at the back of this book.

Caring for a person with a severe mental disorder is likely to require a lot of patience: he or she may have good days and bad days, and tend to make progress in only small steps. A relapse is likely to sap your morale, and it is important that you should be prepared for this. It is a good idea to have an action plan in place before problems arise, and to have discussed it with the general practitioner or local mental healthcare team. If problems arise, contact the general practitioner or mental healthcare team sooner rather than later, because doing so may prevent any problems from getting worse. Remember that your caring role has made you an important source of informa-tion and expertise: learn to rely on your previous experiences and to trust in your judgement. At the same time, try to involve your loved one in making decisions about his or her care.

Sometimes a person with a mental disorder, for example, schizophrenia or bipolar disorder, may fail to recognise that he or she is ill, and so refuse to engage with healthcare services. In particular, he or she may insist that delusions and hallucina-tions are real or may be too paranoid to trust in carers. If your loved one is refusing to engage with healthcare services, you can try to break the prospect of treatment into smaller, more manageable steps, starting with an initial appointment. If possible, give him or her a degree of choice in booking the appointment, and offer to accompany him or her, or to have him or her accompanied.

As progress tends to be made in only small steps, it is easy for you to lose sight of the fact that progress is actually being made. Try to feel positive about your loved one and to gently encourage and facilitate his or her progress. One of the most important things that you can do as a carer is to ensure that your loved one takes his or her medication as prescribed. Be on the lookout for any potential side-effects, and do not hesitate to report them to your general practitioner or local mental healthcare team. Try to establish and maintain a simple daily structure and routine involving regular meal times and sleeping times for your loved one. Gently encourage him or her to attend his appointments with the general practitioner and, if relevant, members of the mental healthcare team and professionals from other services.

Avoid nagging, criticising, telling off, shouting, and arguing. Do not lose sight of the fact that stress is an important predictor of relapse for many mental disorders, and ensure that you are giving your loved one sufficient time and space in which to get better. This can be difficult to achieve, because it is often a carer's instinct to do as much as possible for their loved one, and many carers have unrealistic expectations about the progress that their loved one ought to be making. If you feel that this is an issue for you and the person that you are caring for, speak to the general practitioner or to a member of the mental health-care team about it. Families with these kinds of issues can often be offered educational sessions, stress management, or family therapy: these can all help to reduce stress and can be important and integral parts of the care plan.

Finally, try not to neglect other family members. Brothers and sisters of people with a serious mental disorder, particularly if they are young, may feel that they are not getting their fair share of your attention and become envious and resentful.

Get the practical support that you need

You can obtain an assessment of your needs as a carer by asking your GP to refer you to local Social Services or by referring yourself directly to them. A carer's needs assessment is often helpful in ensuring that your practical needs as a carer are met. You can find out about the carer support services available in your area through Social Services, through a local carers' organisation, or through Carers UK and their dedicated phone line, CarersLine. Such services may include, among other things, help at home, the provision of aids and equipment, break services, and day care. Many carers are reluctant to claim social benefits, either because they have never done so before or because they are put off by the complicated rules and difficult forms. As a carer you play an important role in society, and the benefits that you are entitled to exist to recognise and support that role. Most of these benefits are detailed in Module 46, and you can obtain help in claiming them from your local mental-care team, local Social Services, or voluntary organisations such as Carers UK.

Get the emotional support that you need

Remember that you are not alone as a carer: share your opinions and experiences with the healthcare professionals helping you to look after your loved one, and ask them for help and advice. Conversely, your perspective is invaluable to the healthcare professionals helping you to look after your loved one, so try to accompany him or her to appointments and to participate in discussions about his or her care. Identify someone whom you can talk to on a more personal level – perhaps a relative or a close friend – about your experiences as a carer. Many family members and friends may find it difficult to discuss your caring role, and so underestimate the effort that you are making as a carer. The onus is on you to broach the subject and enlist their help and support. Joining a local carers' group enables you to feel that you are not alone in your carer role, and such a support group can provide a valuable opportunity to learn from the experiences of other carers. Joining a carers' support group can also help you to understand any negative emotions that you may be harbouring, such as guilt, shame, and anger, and to prevent these emotions from affecting the person whom you are caring for.

Look after your physical and mental health

Carers need to care for themselves if they are to care most effectively for a significant other. Many carers come under severe stress and as a result suffer from serious health problems such as heart disease or mental disorder. It is important that you recognise this and take it seriously if you are not to become ill and unable to fulfil your carer role. Use some of the techniques for stress management detailed in Module 13 to reduce your levels of stress, and arrange for an annual health check-up to be carried out by your GP. Make sure that you look after yourself, that you plan and pursue activities that you enjoy, and that you take a break or holiday from caring if you feel that you need one.

Avoid blaming yourself or others

Parents sometimes think that mental disorder in their son or daughter is caused by bad parenting, and fear that they may be to blame for his or her illness. Their feelings of guilt can come to dominate family life, and simply add to the heavy burden already carried by their son or daughter. In the 1940s some psychoanalysts believed that certain mental disorders such as schizophrenia and autism resulted from having a so-called 'refrigerator mother', an emotionally absent and therefore inadequate mother. This theory and other similar theories have never found scientific backing, and have long since been discredited and discarded. In fact, scientific research is quite clear that severe mental disorders such as schizophrenia and bipolar disorder are biological illnesses of the brain.

Parents also sometimes look around for someone else to blame for their son or daughter's illness, such as the general practitioner, the psychiatrist, or even their son or daughter. That they should do so is natural and understandable since it helps them to make sense of the illness of a loved one. Nevertheless, it is important that they remember that the real 'culprit' is usually a biological illness of the brain. They should avoid playing the 'blame game' and instead focus their energies on the challenging journey to recovery.

Like guilt and blame, frustration and anger can be a normal reaction to the illness of a loved one. Parents often have thoughts such as, 'Why did this happen to our family?' or even, 'Why should I even bother? It's too much hard work and, ultimately, it's all going to be for nothing.' Sometimes parents may direct their anger and frustration at their son or daughter, even though they realise that he or she is not to blame for the illness. Unchecked anger only adds to your stress and to that of your son or daughter, and so prevents your family from moving ahead. Although you cannot change the reality of the illness, you can change your reaction to it. Try diffusing your anger by talking about the feelings that underlie it: talk to relatives, friends, healthcare professionals, and other families affected by the same mental disorder. Or else try channelling your anger so that it becomes a force for the good – for example, by motivating you to seek out help for your family.

Your life outside your caring role

Being a carer is often highly stressful and can become all-encompassing. It is important that you think about yourself and your future, because a time may come when you are no longer required to be a carer. As the condition of your loved one improves, he or she may become more independent and in some cases may move out to a place of his or her own. When this happens carers often find themselves lacking in purpose and direction, and unable to adjust to their changed circumstances. For this and other reasons, it is vital that you continue to plan and pursue activities that you enjoy, and that you keep up your life outside your caring role. Many carers are able to be employed in a part-time job, and this can be both a salutatory distraction from the stress of caring and an invaluable source of additional income. Similarly, some carers are able to further their skills, for example, by enrolling on an evening course or on a part-time degree.

Siblings

As parents focus their attention on their mentally ill son or daughter, they run the risk of becoming less available to their other children. These children are also in need of parental attention, not least because they are likely to have been profoundly affected by the illness of their brother or sister. They may be anxious for their family and fearful of developing the illness themselves. Severe mental disorders such as schizophrenia and bipolar disorder often strike in the prime of life, at a time when young people are launching into life – starting college or university, getting a first job, or enjoying an expanding range of activities and social relationships. For this reason, siblings may find it particularly difficult to enjoy their successes while witnessing their ill brother or sister slipping further and further behind. At the same time, they may feel pressured to achieve more so as to 'compensate' for their brother or sister's illness and to avoid adding to the concerns of their afflicted parents.

Siblings should not blame themselves or anybody else for their brother or sister's illness or let it prevent them from enjoying their life outside of the family. By nurturing outside friendships, they may be able to obtain support and talk through difficult feelings such as anger, anxiety, and guilt. Parents need to make a special effort to remember the needs of siblings, and to ensure as far as possible that they are included in family discussions surrounding the illness. Siblings should educate themselves as much as possible about the illness, and also consider joining a carers' support group. Older siblings may be able to play an active role in caring and in due course become an invaluable source of support and respite for their parents. If siblings feel that they are not getting the parental attention that they need, they should not feel afraid or guilty to ask for it.

47 Useful addresses

MIND (National Association for Mental Health)

Website: www.mind.org.uk

The work of mind includes:

- Advancing the views, needs, and ambitions of people with mental health problems.

- Raising public awareness of mental health issues.

- Challenging the discrimination of people with mental health problems and campaigning for their rights.

Through 200 local associations, Mind offers supported housing, crisis helplines, drop-in centres, counselling, befriending, advocacy, employment and training schemes, and other support services.

Through the MIND *info*Line (0845 766 0163 – charged at local rates throughout the UK), Mind offers confidential help on a range of mental health issues and also a special legal service.

Rethink

Website: www.rethink.org

Rethink (formerly the National Schizophrenia Fellowship) offers over 350 services and more than 130 support groups nationally. The range of services includes advocacy, carer support, community support, employment and training, helplines, housing, nursing and residential care, and services dedicated to black and minority ethnic communities. Rethink also produces a quarterly magazine, *Your Voice*, and a range of other publications. You can contact their National Advice Service on 0208 974 6814.

SANE

Website: www.sane.org.uk

The work of SANE includes:

- Campaigning for better services and treatments for people suffering from serious mental illness.

- Undertaking research into the causes of serious mental illness.

- Providing information, crisis care, and emotional support to those experiencing mental health problems and their families and carers through SANELINE (tel: 0845 767 8000 – charged at local rates throughout the UK). SANELINE is open from 1.00 p.m. to 11.00 p.m. every day, including Sundays and Bank Holidays. Calls can be anonymous and their contents are kept confidential.

Making Space

Website: www.makingspace.co.uk

Making Space exists to help all those suffering from mental illness. The current area of operation includes Cheshire, Cumbria, Greater Manchester, Lancashire, Merseyside, Staffordshire, and Yorkshire. Services offered include family and carer support, befriending schemes, day centres, education and training schemes, residential care homes, supported housing schemes, and short breaks and holidays.

MDF The Bipolar Organisation

Website: www.mdf.org.uk

MDF The Bipolar Organisation works to enable people affected by bipolar disorder to take control of their lives. It aims to fulfil this mission by:

- Expanding and developing information services about bipolar disorder.

- Supporting and developing self-help opportunities, including involvement with self-help groups.

- Decreasing discrimination against people with bipolar disorder, and promoting the social inclusion and rights of this group of people.

- Influencing the improvement of treatments and services that improve recovery.

Depression Alliance

Website: www.depressionalliance.org

Depression Alliance is the leading UK charity for people with depression. Its work includes:

- Providing services, including publications, supporter services, local self-help groups, and a pen-friend scheme.

- Carrying out research into depression.

- Campaigning for changes to mental health policy and practices.

- Raising public awareness of depression.

Cruse Bereavement Care

Website: www.crusebereavementcare.org.uk

Cruse Bereavement Care exists to promote the well-being of bereaved people and to enable anyone bereaved by death to understand their grief and cope with their loss.

Relate

Website: www.relate.org.uk

Relate offers help with relationships in the form of advice, relationship counselling, sex therapy, workshops, mediation, consultations, and support face-to-face, by phone, and through their website.

Anxiety UK

Website: www.anxietyuk.org.uk

Anxiety UK is a charity that provides extensive online information on anxiety disorders. Member benefits include therapy services at reduced rates, a member's helpline, and bulletin boards and chat rooms.

No Panic

Website: www.nopanic.org.uk

No Panic is a charity offering support for sufferers of panic attacks, phobias, OCD, generalised anxiety disorder, and benzodiazepine withdrawal. No Panic also offers a telephone helpline (0808 808 0545 – free of charge).

OCD Action

Website: www.ocdaction.org.uk

OCD Action is the largest and longest serving UK charity for people with OCD. The website contains information about OCD and related disorders such as body dysmorphic disorder and compulsive skin picking. Among its many activities, OCD Action organises support groups throughout the UK and offers online support and a telephone helpline (0845 3906232).

beat

Website: www.b-eat.co.uk

beat is the leading UK charity for people with eating disorders and their families, and has a simple vision: Eating Disorders will be Beaten. beat provides helplines for adults and young people, online support, and a UK-wide network of self-help groups to help people beat their eating disorder.

The Sleep Council

Website: www.sleepcouncil.com

The Sleep Council provides useful advice about sleep and about choosing a bed.

Drinkline

Drinkline, the National Alcohol Helpline, can be reached on freephone 0800 917 8282 (Monday to Friday, 9.00 a.m. to 11.00 p.m.). Drinkline is a confidential service that offers information and support to both callers and their relatives and friends.

Alcoholics Anonymous

Website: www.alcoholics-anonymous.org.uk

Alcoholics Anonymous is a spiritually oriented community of alcoholics whose aim is to stay sober and, through shared experience and understanding, to help other alcoholics to do the same, 'one day at a time', by avoiding that first drink. The essence of the programme involves a 'spiritual awakening' that is achieved by 'working the steps', usually with the guidance of a more experienced member or 'sponsor'. Members initially attend daily meetings in which they share their experiences of alcoholism and recovery and engage in prayer or meditation. Alcoholic Anonymous also operate a national 24-hour-helpline (0845 769 7555).

Al Anon

Website: www.al-anonuk.org.uk

Al-Anon offers understanding and support for families and friends of problem drinkers. At Al-Anon group meetings members receive comfort and understanding and learn to cope with their problems through the exchange of experience, strength, and hope. Members learn that there are things that they can do to help themselves and, indirectly, to help the problem drinker.

QUIT

Website: www.quit.org.uk

QUIT's mission statement says that its aim is to provide practical help, advice, and support to all smokers who want to stop. Services include the Quitline (0800 002200), which offers free help and advice, and e-mail counselling (stopsmoking@quit.org.uk).

Cocaine Anonymous

Website: www.cauk.org.uk

Cocaine Anonymous is a fellowship of men and women who share their experience, strength, and hope with each other so that they may solve their common problem and help others to recover from their addiction. The only requirement for membership is a desire to stop using cocaine and all other mind-altering substances.

Narcotics Anonymous

Website: www.ukna.org

Narcotics Anonymous is a non-profit fellowship of men and women for whom drugs has become a major problem. They are recovering addicts who meet regularly to help each other stay clean. The only requirement for membership is the desire to stop using.

The Samaritans

Website: www.samaritans.org.uk

The Samaritans offer a telephone helpline (0845 790 9090 – charged at local rates throughout the UK), which operates 24 hours a day, 7 days a week, every single day of the year. As the Samaritans say:

> 'We're always here to listen. Call us. It doesn't matter who you are – If you are in crisis, despairing or suicidal, contacting us can make all the difference to talk about how you are feeling.

> 'You can speak in total confidence with one of our volunteers about anything that is troubling you. We will not judge you; we will not tell you what to do; but we will try to help you think things through. With Samaritans, you get the time and the space to find a way through.

> 'We will be there for you, to listen with an open mind for as long as you need.'

Papyrus

Website: www.papyrus-uk.org

Papyrus is a voluntary organisation committed to the prevention of young suicide and the promotion of mental health and emotional wellbeing. It provides resources and support for people dealing with suicide, depression, or emotional distress –

particularly teenagers and young adults, as well as a telephone helpline, HOPEline (08000 86 41 51 – free of charge).

CRISIS

Website: www.crisis.org.uk

CRISIS provides help and support to homeless people and people in danger of becoming homeless, so that they can rebuild their lives and escape the cycle of homelessness.

Carers UK

Website: www.carersuk.org

Carers gives so much to society; yet, as a consequence of caring, they can experience ill health, poverty, and discrimination. Carers UK is an organisation of carers fighting to end this injustice. The organisation:

- Mobilises carers and supporters.

- Campaigns for change.

- Transforms understanding of caring.

- Provides information and advice to carers through CarersLine (0808 808 7777 – free of charge).

- Carries out research.

The Royal College of Psychiatrists

Website: www.rcpsych.ac.uk/mentalhealthinformation.aspx

The Royal College of Psychiatrists is the professional and educational organisation for psychiatrists in the UK and Ireland. It produces a range of high-quality publications for the general public, including various leaflets on mental disorders and treatments such as cognitive-behavioural therapy and depot medication.